*How the*
# CIRCULATORY SYSTEM
*Works*

**About the Cover**

The cover is a color-enhanced picture taken by a scanning electron microscope of a cast of one small vein, a small artery, and a number of capillaries. A cast is a model of the space inside vessels (or other hollow organs and tissues); here it is what was left over after the vessels were injected with a special polymeric material and all the tissues were removed by various corrosive means. Be assured this cast was not derived from human tissue.

With the gracious permission of the author and the publisher, this picture is reproduced from Figure 1.11 on page 143 of *Microvascular Corrosion Casting in Scanning Electron Microscopy: Techniques and Applications,* written by S. H. Aharinejad and A. Lametschwandtner and published by Springer-Verlag in 1992.

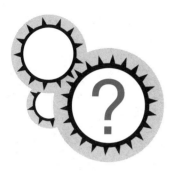

*How the*
# CIRCULATORY SYSTEM
*Works*

By

ROBERT E. MEHLER, MD

Series Editor

LAUREN SOMPAYRAC, PhD

*b*

**Blackwell
Science**

© 2001 by Blackwell Science, Inc.

*Editorial Offices:*
  Commerce Place, 350 Main Street, Malden, Massachusetts 02148, USA
  Osney Mead, Oxford OX2 0EL, England
  25 John Street, London WC1N 2BL, England
  23 Ainslie Place, Edinburgh EH3 6AJ, Scotland
  54 University Street, Carlton, Victoria 3053, Australia
*Other Editorial Offices:*
  Blackwell Wissenschafts-Verlag GmbH, Kurfürstendamm 57, 10707 Berlin, Germany
  Blackwell Science KK, MG Kodenmacho Building, 7-10 Kodenmacho Nihombashi, Chuo-ku, Tokyo 104, Japan

*Distributors:*

*USA*
  Blackwell Science, Inc.
  Commerce Place
  350 Main Street
  Malden, Massachusetts 02148
  (Telephone orders: 800-215-1000 or 781-388-8250; fax
    orders: 781-388-8270)

*Canada*
  Login Brothers Book Company
  324 Saulteaux Crescent
  Winnipeg, Manitoba, R3J 3T2
  (Telephone orders: 204-837-2987)

*Australia*
  Blackwell Science Pty, Ltd.
  54 University Street
  Carlton, Victoria 3053
  (Telephone orders: 03-9347-0300;
  fax orders: 03-9349-3016)

*Outside North America and Australia*
  Blackwell Science, Ltd.
  c/o Marston Book Services, Ltd.
  P.O. Box 269
  Abingdon
  Oxon OX14 4YN
  England
  (Telephone orders: 44-01235-465500;
  fax orders: 44-01235-465555)

Acquisitions: Chris Davis
Development: Julia Casson
Production: Erin Whitehead
Manufacturing: Lisa Flanagan
Director of Marketing: Lisa Larsen
Marketing Manager: Toni Fournier
Cover design by Meral Dabcovich, VisPer
Typeset by Achorn Graphics
Printed and bound by Sheridan Books/Ann Arbor

Printed in the United States of America
00 01 02 03 5 4 3 2 1

The Blackwell Science logo is a trade mark of Blackwell Science Ltd., registered at the United Kingdom Trade Marks Registry

Figure credits: p. 66—Source: Alexander RW, Schlant RC, Fuster V, eds. *Hurst's The Heart.* 1998. Reproduced with permission of the McGraw-Hill Companies.

Library of Congress Cataloging-in-Publication Data

Mehler, Robert E.
  How the circulatory system works / by Robert E. Mehler.
    p. cm. -- (How it works)
  ISBN 0-86542-548-5
  1. Cardiovascular system.   2. Blood--Circulation.   I. Series.

QP101.M456 2000
512.1--dc21

00-039753

To N.A.M., with love.

## *ACKNOWLEDGMENTS*

I must begin by thanking Lauren Sompayrac for making it possible for me to write this book, then for encouraging me to do it, and finally for reading and commenting on it. An additional wonderful benefit sparked by this project has been the great camaraderie that my wife, Nancy, and I now have with Lauren and his wife, Vicki.

Diane Lorenz has done great work in preparing the illustrations. How can anyone so good at her work be so nice?

Everyone at Blackwell Science, Inc., has been very helpful. Among them, Chris Davis, Erin Whitehead, Julia Casson, and Irene Herlihy stand out.

Foremost, I thank my wife, Nancy Aldridge Mehler, for her help. Her expert transcribing and gentle editing made this book possible. She was able to take my hand-printed material -- creatively formed letters and lines in varying geometric patterns -- and turn it into actual blocked paragraphs with lines that read left to right. She is for this book (and for me) a sine qua non.

With such help this book could be perfect. Where it isn't, it is my own doing.

# CONTENTS

CONTENTS

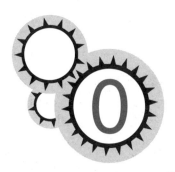

# *HOW TO USE THIS BOOK*

We human beings have always held our circulatory systems in wonder. We saw the human heart as the seat of love and of courage. Our vigor and our ancestry were in our flowing blood. (Now transposed into metaphors, these views nevertheless persist.) And long ago we recognized that the circulation sustains life. As our wonder spurred our interest, we studied our circulatory system and we wrote about what we learned. Today, we continue to study and learn and write at an ever increasing pace, producing many, many books and journals about the circulatory system. Where in that vast array does this small book fit?

This book means to tell a clear, interesting story about the circulatory system -- how its parts work, individually and together, to serve the body. The length of the story has been kept short. It is not exhaustively complete or compulsively detailed. The information presented has been selected to enhance clarity and focus. Yet this book is neither a utilitarian outline nor a cropped summary. The story is enriched by details about basic biologic mechanisms and the nifty ways nature has solved a problem or achieved a result.

This book is organized into lectures rather than chapters, since its style is more conversational than didactic, in keeping with the tone of this series. It is at times lighthearted (but never, I hope, lightweight). The story is fun to tell.

You can read this book, given its length and style, from beginning to end in a few sittings (or even one). I suggest you do that. If something seems murky, mark it and come back to it later. That way you can come to see the circulatory system as a whole and you can get a better sense of its story.

There is some fairly new material in this book, material that shows the direction of present, and probably future, inquiry. With the information provided, both new and old, you will be able to follow much of what is in today's journals and comprehensive textbooks as you pursue your desire to learn more about the circulatory system.

I hope that this small book helps the student of health science to organize and understand this topic; that it reminds the established professional of some of the basic information that is sometimes dimmed by a plethora of details; and that it satisfies the curiosity of the general reader.

# AN OVERVIEW OF THE CIRCULATORY SYSTEM

The human body has by reasonable estimate 75 trillion cells and it prizes all of them. We know this because it provides for each and every cell. To meet this heroic obligation the body uses a quintessential scheme of transport: its own circulatory system.

The circulatory system brings to each individual cell in the very large and very heterogeneous population of cells in the body whatever goods it needs to live and to function, such as nutrients and oxygen, and removes everything it does not need, such as waste products and carbon dioxide. It can meet a wide range of cells' demands and is so self-regulating that there is neither excess nor dearth of goods. It produces neither gridlock nor downtime.

The circulatory system also delivers molecular messages and instructions from other cells, distant or nearby. In case of tissue damage it brings tools for repair and healing to the site. This is a self-sealing circuit; holes can be plugged and fixed. Even new routes can be constructed.

The nature of the components of the circulatory system was obscured for centuries by dogmatic devotion to the writings of the Roman physician Galen. He and his followers held that blood ebbed and flowed from the liver and that the pulse was tied to respiration. It was not until William Harvey made his observations, which he published in 1628 as *De Motu Cordis* (which he dedicated to King Charles I of England, calling him "The Heart of the Commonwealth") that the components of the circulatory system and the path of the circuits were understood and accepted. (Harvey was not able to describe capillaries, though he suspected their existence. That discovery had to wait for the microscope.)

The components of the circulatory system are:

* the heart, the pump;
* the arteries, a series of distributing blood vessels;
* the capillaries, an extensive network of very thin-walled vessels that allows rapid exchange between the body's cells and themselves;
* the veins, a series of collecting blood vessels;
* and the blood, the transport medium that circulates in these channels

The circuitry of the system consists of two main routes connected in series -- that is, one after the other. These are the pulmonary circulation and the systemic circulation. (Note that the word "circulate" comes from the Latin *circulatus,* to form a circle. So we have two essentially circular paths.) The heart is really two pumps in one organ. It pumps unoxygenated blood from its "right heart" to the lungs and receives oxygenated blood from the lungs in its "left heart," which it then pumps into the systemic circulation to the rest of the body. That blood, depleted of oxygen, is returned to the right heart. In the systemic circulation there are separate pathways to target organs and tissues, all arranged in parallel. This means that all the blood goes through the right heart, then the lungs, and then the left heart; but from there it is divided up among all the organs and tissues (except for the lungs).

The heart accomplishes a prodigious amount of work. A Japanese laboratory group calculated that in a lifetime the heart does an amount of work equivalent to raising 16 elephants to the height of Mount Fuji. Converted to Western units, this becomes the equivalent of lifting a herd of 280 cattle from Denver to the height of the Maroon Bells. Either way 240,000,000 kilogrammeters is a lot of work.

The systemic arteries receive the spurts of blood ejected from the beating heart. Serving as a pressure reservoir the arterial system distributes the blood to the capillaries.

Capillaries of the systemic circulation are in very close proximity to cells. No cell is farther than

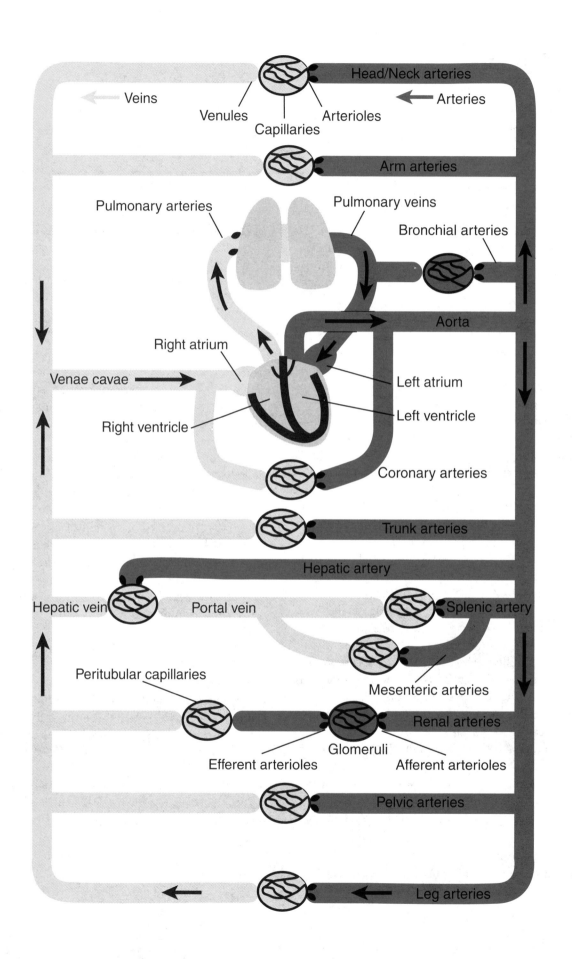

0.1 mm from a capillary. To achieve the needed exchanges, the systemic capillaries have a combined surface area of 600 square meters ($m^2$), somewhat more than the area inside the lines of two tennis courts. The systemic veins collect blood from the capillaries. They act as a volume reservoir and contain most of the blood in the circulatory system. And, of course, they return blood to the heart.

The pulmonary circulation mirrors this pattern -- arteries, capillaries, and veins in sequence. As we will see, this circulation has a number of special features, like the unique role of its capillaries in oxygen and carbon dioxide exchange.

A picture of the overall scheme of the circulation is helpful (see diagram on the left).

Already we catch some curious details about the workings of this system. The circulation to some organs, namely the liver and the kidneys, has two separate capillary networks; the liver and the lungs need (and have) a second blood supply as an oxygen source; and the heart pumps blood to itself.

Let's take this opportunity to review some information that will help us get a grasp on how this whole system works. The concepts of flow, pressure, and resistance and how they are related are key.

- *Flow* refers to how much fluid moves in a given time. For example, we may say the flow from the heart is 5 liters per minute.
- *Pressure* relates to force. It is the force exerted by a liquid (or a gas) on every point of its container. So pressure is force per unit area, like pounds per square inch. (A column of liquid exerts pressure on its base proportional to the height of that column and to the weight or density of the liquid. So pressure can also be expressed as centimeters of water or millimeters of mercury.) A *pressure difference,* also called a pressure *gradient,* may exist between one place and another (between one end of a vessel and the other, for example). This pressure difference is the driving force that causes flow to occur, and it causes that flow to occur from the place of higher pressure to the place of lower pressure.
- *Resistance* is a measure of the hindrance to flow. It is caused by friction between fluid in a vessel and the vessel wall. A longer vessel has more resistance than a shorter one, and a narrower vessel has a *lot* more resistance than a wider one. Also resistance depends on the viscosity of the fluid. *Viscosity* is basically the

"internal friction" in a fluid; it is a measure of how hard it is to get that particular fluid to flow.

In an ideal system flow equals pressure difference divided by resistance.

$$\text{Flow} = \frac{\text{Pressure difference}}{\text{Resistance}}$$

You can increase flow by increasing pressure difference, by decreasing resistance, or by doing both. Similarly you can reduce flow by reducing pressure difference or increasing resistance or both.

Let's apply this concept to the parallel circuit arrangement in the circulatory system (see diagram on following page). Note that in the systemic circulation the pressure difference across the diverse organs and tissues is essentially the same. The total flow through all (not each) of them is the 5 liters per minute the heart pumps. Thus, by changing its resistance each organ can claim more or less of those 5 liters each minute. How much each ends up getting depends also on what its fellow organs are doing with their own resistances.

We must be wary not to confuse analogy with reality. This concept of how pressure, flow, and resistance are related is very useful and affords insight, but it is truly valid only for an ideal hydraulic system. The circulatory system is not made of rigid pipes with fixed dimensions completely filled with a simple solution. Blood vessels have varying amounts of elasticity -- some are even baggy. The amount of fluid (blood) in the system can and does change and when it does the pressure in the system will change also. So when we say, rearranging the previous equation, blood pressure difference equals blood flow times vascular resistance ($P = F \times R$), that is useful but incomplete.

There is often a misconception that circulation to various organs is so competitive that one organ may steal blood from another, causing that organ to be functionally impaired. In fact, the circulatory system is an arrangement of cooperation and balance. It may be true that in some extreme circumstances the demand can exceed the circulatory system's ability to supply. Within a very wide range, however, it is able to supply each organ according to its needs.

The components of the circulatory system fit together and work together, taking advantage of physical forces they create. Thus the circulatory system can fulfill its obligation to meet the needs of each cell in the body, needs that are always present and that often vary.

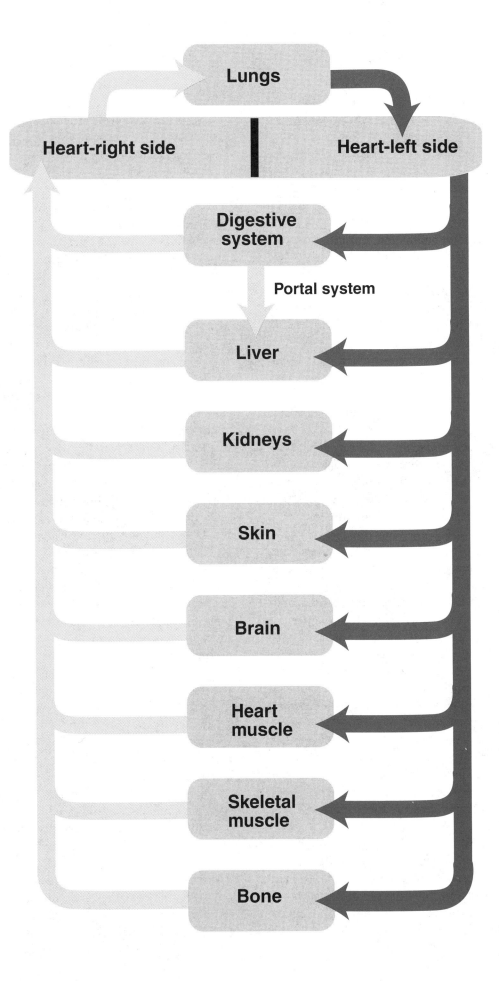

Lungs

Heart-right side | Heart-left side

Digestive system

Portal system

Liver

Kidneys

Skin

Brain

Heart muscle

Skeletal muscle

Bone

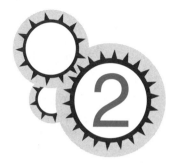

# THE HEART

Would you review that overview?

The circulatory system takes to all the cells in the body what they need and takes from them what they do not need. It does this by providing a constant flow of blood very near each cell. The blood is the transport medium and flows within the confines of the circulatory system. Those confines include the heart, which does the pumping, and the blood vessels—arteries, capillaries, and veins. The heart and blood vessels define two main circuitous routes, one to the lungs and one to the rest of the body. The components of this system work together with extraordinary unity, creating physical forces that result in the proper circulation of blood to every cell.

What is the next lecture about?

The heart -- that pump (two pumps, really) which is automatic, rhythmic, responsive, and lasts a lifetime.

The heart is the perennial choice as the star of the circulatory system. It provides the driving force, the pumping action that moves the blood. Simply seen, it is a hollow muscle that, by contracting, reduces its cavity size and pushes out the blood occupying that cavity. The muscle then relaxes, refilling its hollow interior with blood. It will contract and relax again, and again, and again. This activity is automatic and spontaneous. You do not will your heart to beat. Nor can you consciously instruct it to vary its pumping performance, though when necessary the heart can increase its output many fold.

## FIRST, CELLS

Building an understanding of how the heart muscle works, we begin with the heart muscle cell, the *cardiac myocyte*. The cardiac myocyte has many special characteristics, but it also shares, of course, much of its physiology with the other human cells. It is interesting then to consider not only what is unique about these myocytes but also what features, common to many cells, they have used or adapted to enable them to do their special work.

The *plasma membrane* of the heart muscle cell, its limiting outer boundary, is an example of a common cellular component adorned with special features. This membrane, like that of other cells, is semipermeable. It limits what can pass through. It especially limits molecules that are water soluble.

Most molecules in our bodies are water soluble. Indeed water accounts for 99% of the molecules in us. Yet the plasma membrane has a fatty (*lipid*) middle. In fact, it is a sandwich of two layers of molecules. These molecules are long and skinny. One end, the head, is relatively small and is *hydrophilic*, so it has an affinity for aqueous solutions like those found inside and outside of cells. Extending from the head are two long tails; these tails are fatty acid chains and are *lipophilic*. The heads line up on the surfaces of the plasma membrane (inside and outside) to associate with water, and the tails occupy the middle of the sandwich to avoid water.

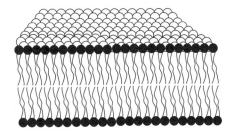

These molecules are not directly attached to each other but their like parts associate (heads with heads, tails with tails). Thus they form a discrete membrane that, because of its lipid center, is a barrier to water soluble molecules. This membrane has fluid-like properties -- that is, some other molecules can float in or on it.

Among the floating molecules is a large number of specific proteins that are embedded in and extend through the membrane. Many of these proteins form special channels or carriers that can allow other molecules, often hydrophilic, to pass through. In addition many of these channel-forming proteins can alter their configurations so that the channel can open and close.

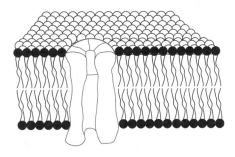

## SOME SHALL PASS

There are two ways molecules can go through the plasma membrane. One is right through the sandwich layers. Lipophilic molecules and small molecules, like oxygen and carbon dioxide, have a relatively easy time taking this route. Or a molecule, most often a hydrophilic one, can go through one of the special channels made of protein, if indeed such a channel exists for that particular molecule and if the channel is open at the time.

There are two reasons molecules go through the plasma membrane at all. The main reason is that particles (atoms or molecules) dissolved in a solution seek a uniform distribution within that solution. Their random motion causes them to move from an area where they are in greater concentration to an area where they are in lesser

concentration. The difference in concentration is called a *concentration gradient* or a *chemical gradient*. The molecular movement is called diffusion. Diffusion occurs quickly over short distances and therefore it is useful to cells because they are so small. For example, given average conditions, molecules we are considering can diffuse a distance of 1 µm (micrometer) in about 0.5 ms (milliseconds). But time of diffusion increases with the square of the distance over which it occurs. So for this same molecule to go 1 mm, it would take over 8 minutes, and it would take 14 hours to go 1 cm. Even cells cannot always rely on diffusion to be quick enough for their needs.

Diffusion results from the constant motion of molecules and is therefore an expression of energy. Whether they are moving in a gas or a liquid, or even in a solid, diffusing molecules seek their most stable spatial arrangement. It takes the addition of opposing energy to counter this process. What this means for us in this discussion is simply that it takes energy to maintain a concentration gradient.

Diffusion can occur through a membrane if that membrane is friendly to the diffusing molecule and allows it to merge in and out of the membrane material. Diffusion can occur through holes or channels in the membrane if these exist. (If a molecule can pass through, the membrane is said to be *permeable* to the molecule, and the molecule is said to be *permeant*.)

A second reason that a molecule would go through a membrane is that it is helped through. There are channels made of protein that transport molecules through the plasma membrane. The most famous of these transport systems has long been called the *sodium pump*. Inside every human cell the concentration of sodium (Na) is lower than it is in the fluid surrounding the cell, the interstitial fluid; potassium (K) is the opposite, higher inside than outside. The plasma membrane is fairly permeable to potassium and is a little bit permeable (usually) to sodium. Yet the concentrations do not equilibrate by diffusion across the membrane because the sodium pump kicks out sodium and brings in potassium. Note that this pumping works against the diffusion tendency and maintains concentration gradients. This takes energy which is supplied by the conversion of adenosine triphosphate (ATP) to adenosine diphosphate (ADP) by the enzyme ATPase. Today this transporter is usually called Na, K–ATPase instead of the more vivid name of sodium pump.

Other transport systems move calcium (Ca) out of cells against a gradient and therefore need energy from ATP. (These are Ca–ATPases). Some other systems exchange sodium for calcium across the plasma membrane, and for reasons later noted, do not directly expend energy in so doing. Calcium-moving devices are very important in muscle cells because calcium plays such a key role in their contractile activity.

Keep in mind a particular difference between the passive diffusion of lipid-soluble molecules through the membrane per se and the passage of some hydrophilic molecules through special channels. The former is an essentially fixed, unchangeable, and nonspecific process. The latter is usually specific and may vary; the channels can change in response to certain stimuli. In short, they can open and close.

## ADDED CHARGE

Until now the several substances mentioned (sodium, potassium, calcium) have been identified only as particles subject to diffusion. But these atoms are *ions* and as such have an electrical charge. That fact adds a whole new force to which they react. Ions obey not only the rules of diffusion but also electromagnetic rules -- opposites ($Na^+$ and $Cl^-$, for example) attract each other and like charges ($H^+$ and $Na^+$, for example) repel each other.

How all cells use this property of ions is remarkable. How cardiac myocytes use it is especially remarkable.

First, consider a relatively simple arrangement. Picture two solutions, separated by a membrane, each with a different concentration of a hypothetical salt XY. Dissolved in water this salt becomes dissociated into ions, $X^+$ and $Y^-$.

If the membrane is equally permeable to $X^+$ *and* $Y^-$ both will pass through and the concentrations on both sides of the membrane will equalize. Nothing new here.

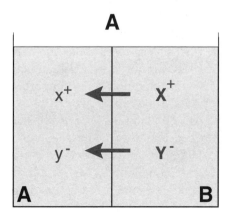

And if the membrane is permeable to *neither* then no movement occurs. Again, nothing new.

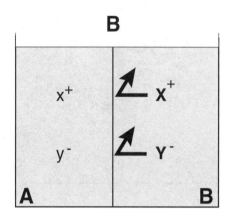

But if the membrane lets $X^+$ through *but not* $Y^-$, then here we do have something new. $X^+$ will diffuse from the side of its greater concentration to the side of its lesser concentration. As it does this, a net positive charge develops on the lesser concentration side, because some $X^+$ ions are there without their $Y^-$ partners. And a negative charge develops on the other side because some $Y^-$ ions are there without their $X^+$ partners. This creates a new kind of gradient, a gradient of charge or an electrical gradient.

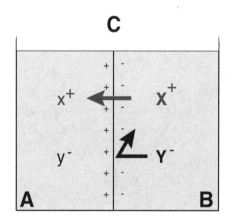

This accumulation of positive charge on one side of the membrane and negative charge on the other creates a force tending to draw $X^+$ back. Two forces, one chemical and one electrical, are now at play. In this case they are acting against each other. At some point they equal each other; an equilibrium is reached, at which point the electrical force bent on retaining X is equal to the chemical force bent on diffusing it. Net movement of $X^+$ stops. Note the compromise: neither side takes all.

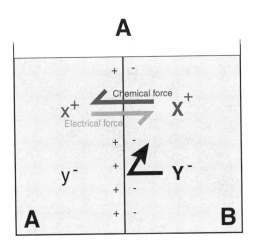

This compromise, this point of equilibrium, can be determined. One simple way is to *measure* it using a voltmeter. (The electrical force is expressed in volts or, in our context, in millivolts.)

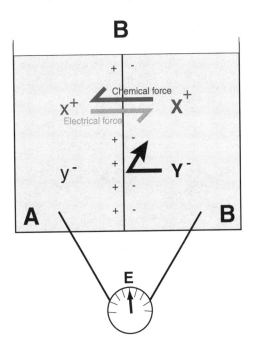

## THE IMPORTANCE OF (BEING) NERNST

The voltage can also be *derived*. Recall that at equilibrium the two forces, chemical and electrical, are equal, though opposite in direction. The chemical force that is due to difference in concentration can be expressed as a ratio of the two concentrations (actually as the logarithm of this ratio) times a constant. The electri-

cal force equals this once the sign is changed (to reflect the opposing direction). So,

$$\text{Electrical force (in volts)} = -K \text{ (constant)} \times \log \frac{[X]B}{[X]A}$$

This is the famous Nernst equation in its simplest form. (Walter Hermann Nernst won the Nobel Prize in chemistry in 1920 for his work in thermodynamics.) Several things about this equation are noteworthy. One is that a relatively big change in the chemical gradient changes the electrical gradient a relatively small amount when equilibrium is reestablished. This is because we are dealing with the logarithm of the ratio. We'll rig the equation a bit and see how this works. Let's say to start that the concentration of $X^+$ is 10 on Side B and 1 on Side A. The units don't matter but we'll call it 10 moles per liter and 1 mole per liter. (You may recall that 1 mole is $6.02 \times 10^{23}$ particles.) So the Nernst equation says,

$$\text{Electrical force} = -K \times \log\left(\frac{10 \text{ mole}/\text{liter}}{1 \text{ mole}/\text{liter}}\right)$$
$$= -K \times 1$$
$$= -K$$

Now we change the concentration of $X^+$ on Side B to 100 moles per liter, increasing it *ten* times. Now at equilibrium the electrical force calculates out to be $-2K$, so we changed it by a factor of only *two*.

A charged particle, an ion, exerts more force because of its "charge" than it does because of its "particle." The movement of only a relatively very small number of charges can create an electrical force capable of countering a large concentration gradient. In fact in our biologic situations, that number of ions is in the range of 1 billionth of those available. The importance of all this is that chemical concentrations are virtually unchanged when ions move to establish an equilibrium.

The Nernst equation is also important because it lets us *analyze* a system in which there is an ion gradient across a membrane. For if we measure the electrical force across the membrane with our voltmeter and it differs from the calculated value (derived from the Nernst equation) for an equilibrium point, we know that the system is not in equilibrium. This means that the electrical and the chemical forces are not equal and are not canceling each other out. Thus ions will tend to flow. The force behind that tendency to flow is the difference between the electrical force (due to the electrical gradient) and the chemical force (due to the chemical gradient). This is called the *driving force* and is a combined electrochemical gradient.

Consider again our solutions of hypothetical ions $X^+$ and $Y^-$. Let's say we calculate that, based on the concentration differences, the electrical potential difference at equilibrium is $-60$ mV. (And don't forget that in our example the membrane is permeable to $X^+$ and not to $Y^-$.)

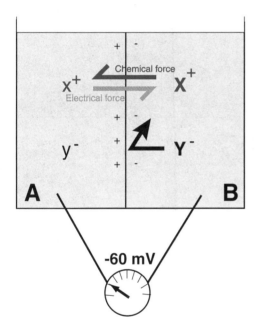

Our voltmeter shows Side B is $-60$ mV compared to Side A. The observed potential difference and the calculated potential difference are both $-60$ mV. The system is in equilibrium: there is no net movement of $X^+$.

Now what if we find with our voltmeter that Side B is $-90$ mV compared to Side A (and the concentrations have not been changed)? First of all, you may ask how this can be. It's easy to see how you can change chemical concentrations of ions, but how do you go about changing electrical gradients? One way would be to use a battery. You could connect one of its two poles to each of the two solutions. How might the body change an electrical gradient? We will come to that. But back to our question: what if the voltmeter reads $-90$ mV?

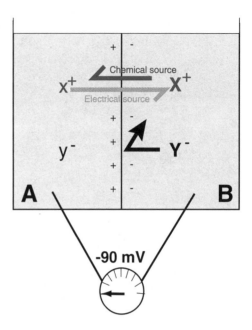

This system is not in equilibrium. There is a 30 mV excess of negative electrical force on Side B, and this will cause $X^+$ to flow toward the negative side, toward Side B. The electrical force is greater than the chemical force.

What if our voltmeter reads $-30$ mV?

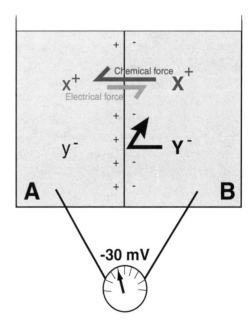

Now there is too little electrical force (by 30 mV) and X will flow toward Side A. Why? Because now the chemical force is greater than the electrical force.

In both instances the systems are seeking to establish the equilibrium point of $-60$ mV.

Let us turn back to cells, and from hypothetical to real. Replace $X^+$ with potassium ($K^+$) and $Y^-$ with negatively charged molecules like proteins, which we will call $P^-$. The cell membrane is permeable to $K^+$, but not to the large negative ions.

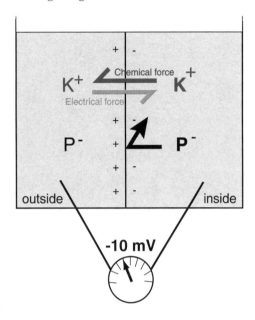

**-10 mV**

This creates a real (though rather small) negative charge inside the cell of about $-10$ mV. (It is the usual convention to compare inside to outside. We chose to compare Side B to Side A in previous pictures to maintain this consistency.)

This is only the beginning of the story. The voltage difference across the plasma membrane of a cardiac myocyte is more like $-90$ mV (again, inside compared to outside). This $-90$ mV electrical potential (called the *resting membrane potential*) is the result of differences in concentrations of several ions -- differences between inside and outside the cell.

Consider $K^+$ first. With this chemical concentration gradient, the electrical potential that would occur across the membrane at equilibrium (as derived by the Nernst equation) would be $-95$ mV. Because the resting

**Ion Concentrations in Millimoles**

|         | Extracellular (outside) | Intracellular (inside) |
|---------|-------------------------|------------------------|
| $K^+$   | 4 mmol                  | 135 mmol               |
| $Na^+$  | 145 mmol                | 10 mmol                |
| $Ca^{2+}$ | 2 mmol                | $10^{-4}$ mmol         |

membrane potential is in fact $-90$ mV, there is a small force tending to push $K^+$ out of the cell.

Now look at sodium ($Na^+$). Here the situation is quite remarkable. Because $Na^+$ concentration is higher outside than inside the cell, equilibrium would not be reached until the electrical potential was $+70$ mV (inside $+70$ mV compared to outside).

**A**

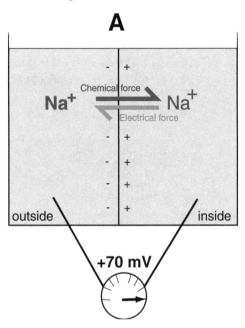

**+70 mV**

What happens when the membrane potential is $-90$ mV? Note that here the driving force trying to push $Na^+$ into the cell is the total of 160 mV -- all the way from $-90$ mV to $+70$ mV.

**B**

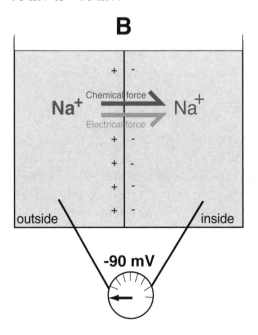

**-90 mV**

The electrical and chemical forces are not opposing each other but rather are in the same direction. Calcium ($Ca^{2+}$) is even more striking with an equilibrium potential of $+132$ mV.

Each of these ions seeks its equilibrium point. So why is the resting membrane potential ($-90$ mV) so close to what $K^+$ seeks ($-95$ mV) and so far from what $Na^+$ and $Ca^{2+}$ seek? Because the plasma membrane is, in the resting state, much more permeable to $K^+$ than it is to $Na^+$ or $Ca^{2+}$.

This is a major take-home point. The ion that the plasma membrane lets pass through most easily (for which the membrane is most permeable) has the most clout. Its equilibrium point is most expressed.

The resting membrane potential of a cardiac myocyte is $-90$ mV, a bit less than the $-95$ mV that $K^+$ is seeking, because $Na^+$ and $Ca^{2+}$ do have a little influence. The plasma membrane is very slightly permeable to them in the resting state.

The 5 mV difference between the resting membrane potential and the $K^+$ equilibrium point does tend to push some $K^+$ out of the cell. Why doesn't this deplete intracellular $K^+$ and lower its intracellular concentration? Because the sodium pump pushes $Na^+$ out and brings $K^+$ into the cell, and spends energy in the form of ATP to do it. The potassium concentration gradient and the resting membrane potential are maintained.

## POLAR(ITY) EXPEDITIONS

Now the stage is set for action. But first, let's digress a minute to answer a question posed earlier, and to make another take-home point. A cell can change the electrical potential across its membrane by changing the permeability of one of its ions. And it can change that permeability by opening or closing that ion's specific channels.

Back to the action. Events occur that result in the contraction of the heart muscle cell. The first of these events is a sudden reduction in membrane potential from $-90$ mV to $-65$ mV. A reduction in membrane potential is really a reduction in the amount of charge difference across the membrane -- that is, a reduction in polarity. It is called *depolarization*. An increase in polarity is called *hyperpolarization*. Suffice it to say for now that this depolarization, from $-90$ to $-65$mV, happens.

And it happens suddenly. (What makes it happen we will consider later.) At $-65$ mV membrane potential, sodium channels -- those plasma membrane channels that can allow $Na^+$ through -- begin to open up. The new membrane potential of $-65$ mV is in fact the signal for them to open. For this reason they are called *voltage-dependent channels*. This means that the plasma membrane is now permeable to $Na^+$ and the equilibrium potential of sodium gets to be expressed.

As the membrane is further depolarized, more and more voltage-dependent sodium channels open until the membrane potential reaches about $+20$ mV, when they close. This opening and closing of these sodium channels happens very quickly. The channels themselves are often referred to as "fast sodium channels." This burst of membrane permeability to sodium causes the membrane potential to change, quite suddenly, from $-90$ mV to $+30$ mV. When the sodium channels close, potassium resumes its role as the dominating permeant ion and the resting membrane potential is reestablished. The plasma membrane is *repolarized*.

The up and down spike in membrane potential is called an *action potential* and is triggered by the plasma membrane reaching its threshold potential of $-65$ mV.

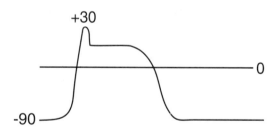

Cells that can generate an action potential are considered "excitable."

One characteristic of an action potential is that it is propagated very quickly over the whole cell surface. That is because if one small area of plasma membrane reaches its threshold potential and has an action potential triggered, that $+30$ mV area sits next to a $-90$ mV area and local current flow occurs. This will reduce the amount of polarity of that adjacent area. The membrane potential becomes less negative, reaches its threshold of $-65$ mV, and bingo, more action potential.

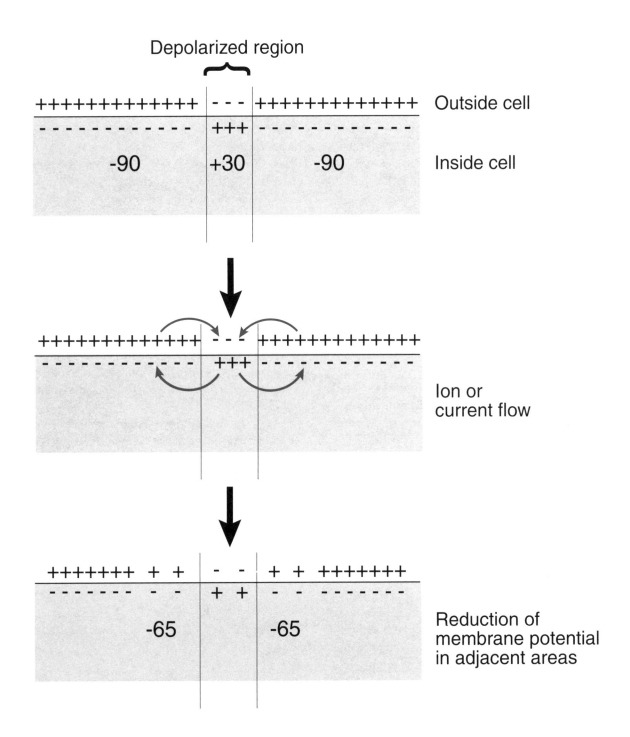

Depolarized region

++++++++++++ - - - ++++++++++++++    Outside cell
- - - - - - - - - - - - +++ - - - - - - - - - - -
-90    +30    -90    Inside cell

++++++++++++++ - - - ++++++++++++++
- - - - - - - - - - - - - +++ - - - - - - - - - -    Ion or
current flow

++++++  +  +  - -  +  +  ++++++
- - - - - -  - -  +  +  - -  - - - - - -
-65    -65    Reduction of
membrane potential
in adjacent areas

Again, how the first threshold potential was reached will come later.

Is it the action potential that makes the myocyte contract? Well, not quite. The real link between the action potential and contraction is calcium ($Ca^{2+}$).

Small tubules (called T-tubules), which are extensions of the plasma membrane, dip down, mak-

ing deep pits on the surface of the cardiac cell. These lie close to the cell's endoplasmic reticulum. (You remember the endoplasmic reticulum is the series of membranous compartments in cells' cytoplasm. In muscle cells this is called sarcoplasmic reticulum -- from the Greek σαρξ meaning "flesh.") The sarcoplasmic reticulum is very rich in $Ca^{2+}$, most of which is loosely bound to protein.

## KUDOS TO CALCIUM

As an action potential rapidly sweeps over a cardiac cell, it also then dives into the cell via the T-tubules. There are voltage-regulated $Ca^{2+}$ channels in the plasma membrane, including that of T-tubules. With depolarization, $Ca^{2+}$ channels are opened and extracellular $Ca^{2+}$, following its electrochemical gradient, comes into the cytoplasm. This is not yet enough calcium to lead to contraction. This influx of $Ca^{2+}$ instead is a trigger to release a bigger burst of calcium from the sarcoplasmic reticulum. With this release of $Ca^{2+}$ from the sarcoplasmic reticulum, the level of $Ca^{2+}$ in the cell cytoplasm increases 10 to 100 times. This is enough $Ca^{2+}$ to ignite contraction.

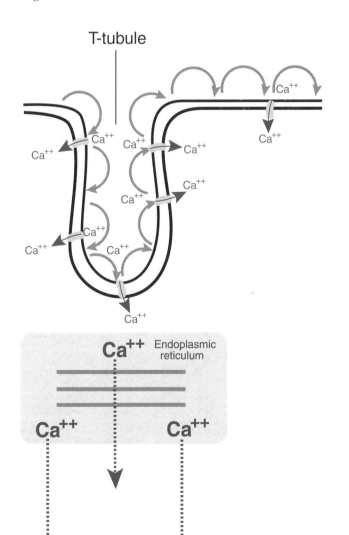

So the cascade of events so far is as follows: resting membrane potential → threshold membrane potential → action potential → influx of $Ca^{2+}$ from outside cell → release of $Ca^{2+}$ from sarcoplasmic reticulum → muscle contraction.

Just as increased $Ca^{2+}$ in the cytoplasm leads to myocyte contraction, reduction of $Ca^{2+}$ causes relaxation. As the membrane repolarizes, plasma membrane calcium channels close and calcium influx from outside the cell stops. The sarcoplasmic reticulum is no longer signaled to release calcium. Now the calcium pumps in the sarcoplasmic reticulum bring calcium back into that compartment. These pumps require energy supplied by ATP. They are activated or "primed" by a protein phospholamban. (We will meet phospholamban again later.) There are also energy-requiring $Ca^{2+}$–ATPases ($Ca^{2+}$ pumps) in the plasma membrane. These help reestablish intracellular calcium levels by moving calcium back out of the cell. These pumps are stimulated by another protein, calmodulin, when calcium binds to it. (More on calmodulin later.)

Another important transport system used to move calcium out of the cell through the plasma membrane is the sodium/calcium exchanger. Here one calcium ion leaves the cell in exchange for three sodium ions that enter the cell. These sodium ions are then pumped out by the sodium pump. The exchanger itself does not directly require ATP. It takes advantage of sodium's gradient to extrude calcium from the cell. However, there is an ultimate energy expense because the sodium has to be pumped out. Note that this relaxation phase is not passive but is an energy-consuming active process.

## BRIDGING AND SLIDING

What is it that the $Ca^{2+}$ ions act on that results in contraction or shortening of the cell? What is the tiny machine, responding to $Ca^{2+}$, that changes chemical energy into mechanical energy?

Inside the heart muscle cell, which is much longer than it is wide, are bundles of tiny strands, called myofibrils, which lie along the cell's axis. Each myofibril is a series of basic contractile units, the sarcomeres, which are placed end to end. Each sarcomere is supported by a protein scaffolding that helps support and align its elements. It is this precise lining up of each fibril's elements in the cardiac myocyte that allows them to show up under a microscope as bands or striations, thus classifying cardiac muscle as striated muscle. Each sarcomere is a cylinder in which two kinds of filaments -- described as thick and thin -- overlie each other. The thin filaments are attached to cytoskeletal discs that, when lined up, form a Z-line. The distance between two Z-lines measures the sarcomere length. M-lines are created by other cytoskeleton proteins that hold the thick filaments in line. When thin filaments slide over thick filaments, the sarcomere shortens.

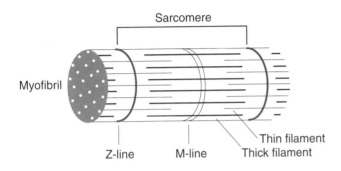

The thin filaments contain two major proteins, actin and tropomyosin. Actin is double-stranded and made up of globules strung together; tropomyosin molecules are rod-shaped. These proteins are arranged in strands that twist on each other. Bound to the tropomyosin is another protein, troponin.

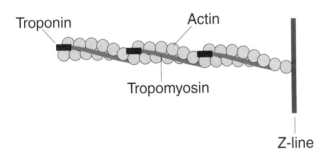

The thick filaments are made of a larger protein, myosin. Each myosin molecule has two tails and two globular heads.

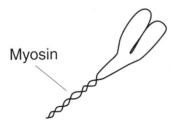

The tails twist around each other and, along with tails of other myosins, form the backbone of each thick filament.

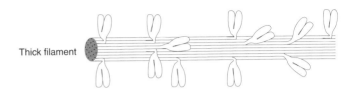

The heads of these myosin proteins stick out and lie adjacent to the thin filaments.

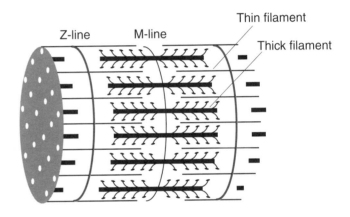

These filaments, thick and thin, are all arranged neatly in a hexagonal pattern, with two thin filaments for every thick filament.

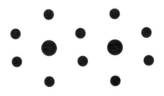

This is a cross-sectional picture of just two myosin thick filaments with their neighboring thin filaments. Myosin heads are not shown. Note that while there are *two* thin filaments for each thick filament, each thick filament has access to *six* thin filaments.

The myosin heads can form connections, or crossbridges, with the actin of the thin filaments. Each head, linked with actin at 90 degrees, can bend 45 degrees, pulling the actin over the thick filament. It can then detach and do it again, or it can stay detached.

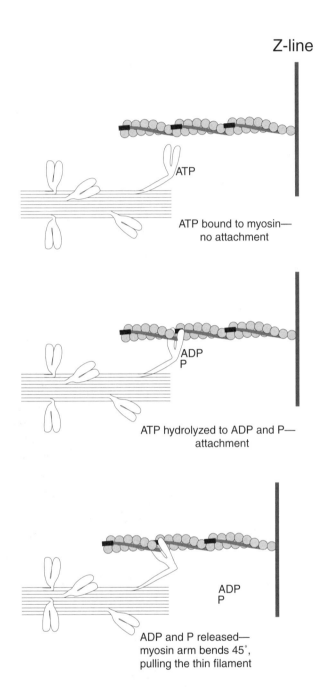

Z-line

ATP

ATP bound to myosin—
no attachment

ADP
P

ATP hydrolyzed to ADP and P—
attachment

ADP
P

ADP and P released—
myosin arm bends 45°,
pulling the thin filament

How does that work? When $Ca^{2+}$ rises in the cell (remember, chiefly from the sarcoplasmic reticulum) it binds to troponin. This causes a shift in structure that uncovers binding sites on actin for the myosin head. Meanwhile, ATP has bound to the myosin head. Myosin acts as ATPase, converting ATP to ADP and phosphorus (P), both of which are still attached to the myosin head. In this configuration there is increased affinity of myosin for actin.

With this increased affinity of myosin for actin

and with the uncovering of binding sites on actin by $Ca^{2+}$, crossbridging occurs. Now ADP and P are released and now the real mechanical event occurs: the myosin head–actin-binding site shifts from 90 degrees to 45 degrees, causing the filaments to slide over each other shortening the sarcomere by 10 nm. (One nanometer is 1 billionth of 1 m.) Now ATP again binds to the myosin head, which reduces the affinity for actin, and the crossbridge detaches. Crossbridging cycles can repeat as long as $Ca^{2+}$ is sufficiently high.

Each thick filament of myosin has 300 to 400 myosin heads (i.e., potential crossbridges) and each sarcomere has many thick filaments, and each myofibril has many sarcomeres, and each muscle cell has many myofibrils, and the heart has many cells. The number of crossbridging events for each heartbeat is enormous.

Heart muscle cells need a lot of ATP because they do a lot of work. The crossbridging cycles consume the most energy, but the needs of other processes are considerable. The ion pumps that maintain ion gradients between action potentials and that restore ion gradients after action potentials are ATP dependent. Synthetic and metabolic processes, like intracellular protein production, also require energy.

Although some skeletal muscle fibers can derive ATP from the breakdown of glucose without oxygen at least for a short time, cardiac myocytes cannot. They require oxygen for their production of ATP from both glucose and fatty acids.

This means that heart muscle cells need a rich continuous blood supply to bring oxygen, and they need many mitochondria to produce enough ATP to meet immediately their demands. Mitochondria, you recall, are the cells' organelles in which, through an oxidative process, energy derived from metabolism is packaged as ATP.

## FROM CELLS TO TISSUE

The myriad cardiac myocytes have a unique arrangement as they form heart muscle tissue. They have branches along their long axes allowing each cell to meet several others end to end. The places where they meet are *intercalated discs*, which contain *gap junctions*. These are special junctions that offer very low resistance to the transmission of an action potential from a connecting cell, facilitating the rapid conduction of the action potential from one cell to the next. Just as the action potential spreads across this tissue, so does an episode of contraction and relaxation.

## FROM TISSUES TO ORGAN

Let us now begin our look at the heart as an organ. How does this tissue, made up of cells and capable of nearly simultaneous contraction and then relaxation, arrange itself to create blood flow? What is the design of this pump?

First we will look at the components of the pump and how they are arranged. Later we will consider how these components are coordinated.

The human heart has four chambers, two atria above and two ventricles below. One of each comprises the right pump and one of each the left pump. These two pumps beat simultaneously. The "right heart" receives unoxygenated blood from the general circulation and pumps it via the pulmonary artery to the lungs where it takes up oxygen.

The "left heart" receives oxygenated blood from the lungs via the pulmonary veins and pumps it into the general circulation supplied by the largest artery, the aorta. The atria are smaller than the ventricles and have thinner walls. Each atrium has a small appendage called an auricula (because of its ear-like

shape). The atria are separated from each other by a wall or septum, which is relatively thin.

The ventricles are separated by a muscular septum. The muscular walls around the ventricles are thicker than the atrial walls. The left ventricle is thickest of all, because it works in a higher pressure system than the right ventricle. The continuum of muscle fibers in the ventricles sweeps from the top down to the apex of the heart. These fibers are arranged so that with contraction not only does the heart's circumference decrease but its longitudinal axis shortens.

The right heart lies rightward and mostly toward the front, and the left heart lies leftward and mostly toward the back. The heart itself is shaped like a blunt cone and is about the size of the fist of the person to whom it belongs (or, as stated in *Grey's Anatomy*, "in whose bosom it beats"). It looks very little like the valentine heart shape ♡. (Actually, among body parts, that depiction probably best represents the prostate gland.)

Each atrium is separated from its ventricle by a valve (atrioventricular valve); the one on the right is called the tricuspid and on the left is the mitral. The tricuspid has three leaflets. The mitral valve has two and is sometimes called the bicuspid valve. (It looked to some past anatomist like a miter -- a bishop's hat.) Each valve is a tough ring with its leaflets attached to it. Each opens in one direction only: into the ventricle. Thus the

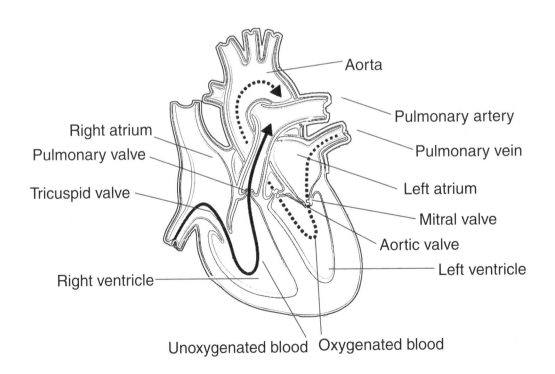

Aorta

Pulmonary artery

Pulmonary vein

Right atrium

Pulmonary valve

Tricuspid valve

Left atrium

Mitral valve

Aortic valve

Left ventricle

Right ventricle

Unoxygenated blood    Oxygenated blood

direction of blood flow is established, from atrium to ventricle. The atrioventricular valve leaflets are tethered to their respective ventricular walls to prevent backflow when they are closed.

Between each ventricle and its receiving artery (pulmonary artery on the right, aorta on the left) is a valve, called pulmonary and aortic, respectively. When open, these valves allow flow out of their respective ventricles. Each of these valves is composed of a ring to which are attached three delicate but very strong cusps, which are not tethered. When the valve is closed, each cusp abuts on its two neighbors to create a tight closure without backflow. These valves are sometimes called semilunar valves because of the half-moon shape of each cusp when viewed from the side.

Even though the heart has blood coursing through it, it requires its own blood supply, its own system of arteries and veins. This is made clear by the fact that the heart is apt to weigh 300 grams and have a left ventricular muscle thickness of 10 to 12 mm. Thus, its size precludes the possibility of its receiving adequate oxygen and nourishment from the diffusion of oxygen and nutrients from the blood in its chambers. Recall not only the heart's high immediate demand for oxygen, but also the slow speed of diffusion over "long" distances.

The coronary arteries provide blood to the heart. There are two main arteries, the left coronary and right coronary, and both arise from the aorta just above the aortic valve.

- The right coronary artery supplies the right atrium and ventricle, and the atrioventricular node (more on that later), and the posterior surface of the left ventricle.
- The left coronary artery divides into the left anterior descending and the circumflex, creating two major pathways. The left anterior descending artery supplies the front of the left ventricle and much of the interventricular septum. The circumflex supplies the left atrium and the left lateral ventricle.

These arteries, of course, divide into smaller and smaller branches. These feed into capillaries, which in turn drain into small veins that become large veins. The veins follow roughly the distribution of the major arteries. The veins finally join into a single trunk, the coronary sinus, which empties into the right atrium.

On the outside of the heart is a thin protecting layer of tissue (not muscle) called the epicardium (*epi*, upon). Lining the inside of the heart is a thinner

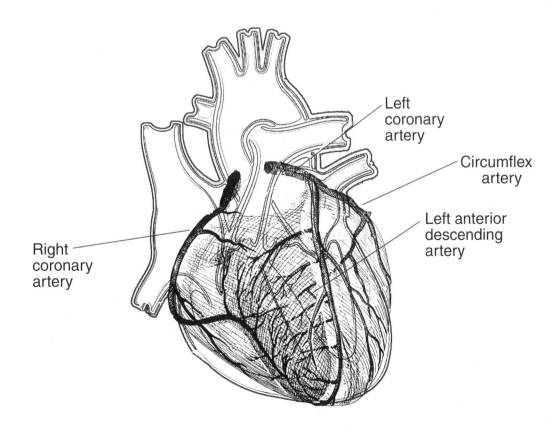

Left coronary artery

Circumflex artery

Left anterior descending artery

Right coronary artery

layer of tissue, the endocardium (*endo,* within). The muscle tissue in between is the myocardium. The pericardium (*peri,* around) is the fibrous sack in which the heart sits.

## GETTING THE MESSAGE OUT

With each heartbeat the atria contract first. Then, after a slight delay, the ventricles contract. The chambers then relax, refilling with blood. What initiates this sequence and how is it coordinated?

A very special small lump of tissue -- the sinoatrial (SA) node -- lies just at the junction of the right atrium with the superior vena cava, one of the two large veins that empty into it. The SA node, which is about 8 mm long and 2 mm wide, is the pacemaker of the heart. Here begins the action potential that spreads through the heart, signaling it to beat.

The cells of the SA node have special physiologic features that allow them spontaneously to create an action potential. It can be said that they create their own excitement. Until now all the heart cells we have considered have required an outside stimulus to raise their resting membrane potential to their threshold potential. Finally we are seeing how that first threshold potential in each heartbeat comes about.

We can appreciate what is special about how the SA node cells work if we first review and expand on the sequence of the action potential found in most myocardial cells. These are known as fast response action potentials. Recall that most myocardial cells have a resting membrane potential of $-90$ mV. When this is suddenly raised to about $-65$ mV a threshold is crossed and membrane sodium channels are opened. There is a rapid depolarization, changing the membrane potential to $+30$ mV. This change opens calcium ($Ca^{2+}$) channels, allowing calcium to enter the cell, which in turn triggers the cascade of events that results in contraction. The calcium channels stay open longer (that is, they inactivate more slowly) than the sodium channels. Thus, there is a plateau period of continuing influx of $Ca^{2+}$ into the cell, during which the membrane potential remains positive. During much of this plateau the membrane potassium channels are closed (at least more are closed than usual). As calcium channels close and potassium channels open, the resting membrane potential is reestablished and remains

constant -- until another depolarizing event from outside the cell raises the membrane potential to threshold level.

It all looks like this:

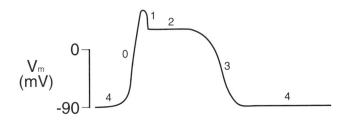

**A fast response action potential**

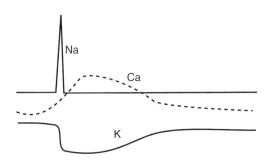

**Simultaneous relative permeances of ions involved**

The phases of the action potential are numbered.

0. Rapid depolarization -- a combination of resting membrane potential raised to threshold and the following sudden influx of sodium ($Na^+$).
1. Notch of repolarization caused by a brief outflow of $K^+$ before its channels close.
2. The plateau.
3. Repolarization.
4. Resting membrane potential.

All this is characteristic of fast response action potentials. In a relatively few cardiac cells there is another kind of action potential called *slow response.* SA node cells are in the slow response camp. Characteristically in these cells the resting membrane potential is less negative; there is little or no plateau, and there is no phase 1.

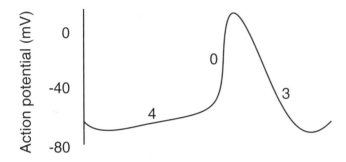

But the pacemaker cells have an additional special feature. Look at phase 4. Note that there is a slow depolarization occurring and the threshold, at which an action potential is triggered, is reached spontaneously. This slow rise in membrane potential is the result of "leaking" of all three ions, $Na^+$, $K^+$, and $Ca^{2+}$. The inward currents or movements of $Na^+$ and $Ca^{2+}$ cause gradual depolarization or drift of the membrane potential toward the threshold, and these are opposed by the outward leak of $K^+$ ions. But that opposing flow of $K^+$ gradually decreases throughout phase 4. Thus, the automatic depolarization proceeds in these SA node cells until the threshold potential is reached and an action potential is generated.

This action potential is conducted throughout the right atrium from cell to cell and then across to the left atrium and over it as well. The speed of conduction is about 1 meter/second.

This atrial excitation wave does not go directly to the ventricles. There is in fact a barrier between the atria and the ventricles, complete except for another specialized nest of cells called the atrioventricular (or AV) node. This track is about 22-mm long and runs from the lower right side of the interatrial septum downward to merge with the upper portion of the Bundle of His, another track of specialized fibers that takes the action potential to the ventricles. In the AV node there is slower conduction, with the impulse traveling at about 0.05 meter/second. (This slow conduction in the AV node creates a time delay, ensuring that the ventricles contract after the atria.) The Bundle of His passes down the right side of the interventricular septum for about 1 cm and then divides into two branches, a left and a right bundle branch. The larger left bundle branch penetrates the septum to reach the left ventricle where it too divides, into an anterior fascicle and a posterior fascicle. The right bundle branch proceeds down the right side of the septum to the right ventricle. Each of

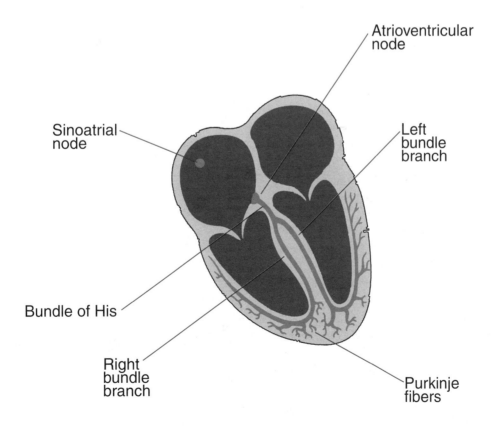

these three main divisions ultimately subdivides into a network of conducting fibers called Purkinje fibers, which spread out over the inner surfaces of both ventricles. These are thick cells able to carry the action potential very rapidly, up to 4 meters / second.

You well might worry about this system with its rather herky-jerky method of sending out the action potential. It has fairly rapid conduction in the atrium, is slow in the AV node, and ultimately is very fast in the ventricles. What is to keep that wave of electrical activity from moving back and forth across the ventricle or looping back up to the AV node and from there to the atria, all creating chaos rather than rhythm? Your worries can be allayed by what is called the refractory period.

The *refractory period* is the time during the action potential -- essentially from the beginning until well along in phase 3 -- when a cell cannot develop another action potential. In fact, a cell is not fully excitable until it has been completely repolarized. Therefore, as a rule, once a wave of depolarization (an action potential) has swept across the heart, both the conducting fibers and the myocytes are briefly dormant, so only one beat can occur at a time.

You may also wonder what happens if the SA node fails to do its job. Does the heart, without its pacemaker, just stop beating? It turns out that a number of cells, chiefly other atrial cells, AV node cells, and Purkinje cells, also are capable of spontaneous depolarization (only at a slower rate than SA nodal cells) and can take over to pace the heart if the SA node fails.

Here then is the heart's conduction system, the path by which it generates, propagates, and coordinates the message to its muscle cells to contract. Combined in one system are two key features of the beating heart: it is automatic (able to initiate its own beat) and it is rhythmic (able to repeat regularly that beat).

Incidentally, it is this electrical activity sweeping over the heart that, when recorded, yields an electrocardiogram (ECG). From this record one can answer a number of questions, such as: Is the SA node doing its job? Is there any problem with the path over which the electrical activity is conducted? Is there a part of the heart that is not, for some reason, participating normally?

Up to this point we have looked at what makes the heart beat and why it beats spontaneously and regularly. We have not yet gotten to how the heart really functions as a pump.

## THE CARDIAC CYCLE

How is it that beating means pumping? This question is best answered both with a graph and with a narrative in which we take a look at the cardiac cycle, describing step by step what goes on during contraction (emptying) or *systole,* and relaxation (filling) or *diastole.*

We will first look at the left heart pump, and then note what is going on virtually simultaneously in the right heart.

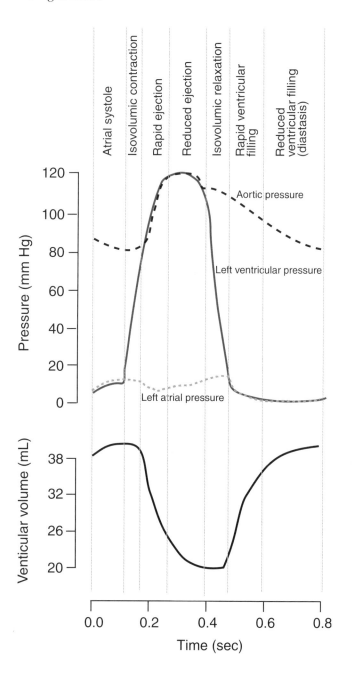

Even though the atria contract first, let us begin with the power stroke of the heart, the ventricular systole. As left ventricular contraction starts, the mitral valve and aortic valve are both closed. Pressure increases in the ventricle until it just equals the pressure in the aorta. This is called isovolumic (same volume) contraction. As the ventricular pressure goes still higher it exceeds the aortic pressure. Now the aortic valve opens and blood is pumped into the aorta. This is the ventricular ejection phase. At first there is a brief time of rapid ejection, then a longer period of reduced rate of ejection. During the rapid ejection phase there is a sharp rise in ventricular and aortic pressures, a rapid decrease in left ventricular volume, and large aortic blood flow. During the reduced ejection phase there is decreasing ventricular and aortic pressure but still there is flow from the ventricle into the aorta. As pressure in the ventricle decreases it is exceeded by aortic pressure and the aortic valve closes. Again there is a brief period when the mitral and aortic valves are both closed and during which ventricular pressure is falling. This is the first phase of diastole and is called isovolumic relaxation. When the ventricular pressure falls below that of the left atrium, the mitral valve opens and the rapid filling phase occurs. This is when most of ventricular filling occurs. With the fall in atrial and ventricular pressure there is a marked increase in left ventricular volume. There follows a period of slower left ventricular filling (often called diastasis). It is only at the end of this phase that atrial systole occurs, with variable contribution to ventricular volume (less contribution with slow heart rate, more with rapid heart rate). At the very onset of left ventricular contraction, left ventricular pressure exceeds left atrial pressure and the mitral valve closes.

Atrial contraction optimizes ventricular filling. That atrial contraction occurs first is thanks to the AV node's delaying ventricular excitation so that the atrium has time to make its contribution and is not opposed by the contracting ventricle. Recall, however, that most ventricular filling occurs before the atria contract. The beating of the atria promotes flow to the ventricles but it is not a necessary contribution at most levels of cardiac performance.

Note that during diastole, pressure in the aorta is falling as runoff continues to occur into the downstream vessels.

The same pattern occurs in the right heart, only with lower pressures.

## LISTENING

When you listen to the heart, you usually hear two sounds, traditionally described as "lub-dup." The first sound, lub, is generated by the closing of the AV valves, thus signaling onset of systole. The second sound, dup, is the result of the semilunar valves closing and occurs at the beginning of diastole. In fact, if you listen closely to the second heart sound you may note that it is split -- that is, it has two components. This is because the aortic valve closes slightly before the pulmonary valve. This split is more likely to be audible during inspiration when the difference in closing times increases.

## WORK, WORK, WORK

Do you remember all that work the heart does -- all those kilogram-meters (or large animals raised to mountain heights)? The work of any pump can be calculated by multiplying the pressure against which it pumps times the volume it moves. Why is that? Because kilograms/$m^2$ (pressure) $\times$ $m^3$ (volume) = kilogram-meters (work). The heart's work each beat then is

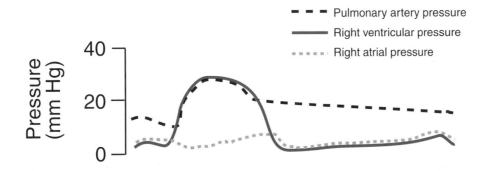

approximately equal to average aortic pressure times the amount of blood pumped with that beat.

One would think that there would be a good correlation between the work done by the heart and how much oxygen it uses, because oxygen use is a measure of energy expended. But all work is not equal. If heart work is increased by raising aortic pressure, the heart needs more oxygen (energy) than if an identical increase in work is effected by increasing the volume of blood pumped. This means that it is harder, more energy demanding, for the heart to do "pressure work" than to do "volume work."

Overall, given the usual resting blood pressure and cardiac output, the heart's work efficiency rating is 18%. That means the ratio of work accomplished to energy used is 0.18. In designing the heart, as in designing so many of her works, Nature preferred cleverness to efficiency. (More on this later.)

We have come a long way in understanding the heart as a pump -- a pulsatile, self-activating, unidirectional pump. This would be fine if all we needed was a device that would put out a fixed amount -- say, 5 liters a minute. However the body's demand for blood, with its oxygen and nutrients, varies. So sometimes more blood has to be pumped, sometimes less. Of note is that some human hearts can increase their output per minute by six to seven times during exercise. The amount of blood returning to the heart to be pumped and the pressure in the arterial system into which the blood is sent may also vary.

Recall also that the heart is really two pumps that, though they are wrapped in one organ, are separate. They are arranged in series, one after the other, in the flow scheme and therefore must maintain virtually equal outputs. If the right heart pumped more than the left heart, blood would pool in the lungs. If the left heart pumped more than the right heart, blood would pool in the general circulation.

All these needs for the heart to adapt and vary its pumping action are met by a variety of control mechanisms. Some of these are found in the heart itself (intrinsic controls) and some originate outside the heart (extrinsic controls).

## INSIDERS

The heart's built-in adapters (intrinsic controls) are especially fascinating because they are so tidy. Re-

call that at the end of diastole the ventricle is filled with blood, an amount that is called the end-diastolic volume. This is also referred to as *preload* and it is the workload (essentially "volume" work) impressed on the heart *just before* contraction begins. This preload causes some stretch on the muscle fibers of the ventricle, filled as it is.

Now let us say that for some reason there is an increase in the amount of blood coming to the right atrium. For example, if a man lies down and raises his legs, the amount of blood that had been distending the leg veins while he was standing is released. This increase in blood, on reaching the right ventricle, increases the preload, and increases the stretch on the right ventricle myocytes. This causes greater contraction of the myocytes, which translates into increased force of contraction of the right ventricle to meet the increased load. Now when the increased output of the right ventricle reaches the left heart, the same thing happens, resulting in increased force of contraction and causing greater left ventricular volume to be pumped out. Thus, not only can more or less blood returning to the heart be handled appropriately, but the output of the two pumps can be balanced. This ability of the heart to respond to changes in the length of myocardial fibrils is called the Frank-Starling mechanism, after Otto Frank and Ernest Starling who independently described it about a hundred years ago.

What causes the stretching of a cardiac myocyte to make it contract with more force? The chief reason lies in the sarcomere. As the sarcomere is stretched (up to a limit of about 2.2 μm), its sensitivity to $Ca^{2+}$ increases. Here again $Ca^{2+}$ is the key. There is a limit to this mechanism, of course. Beyond sarcomere length of 2.2 μm the force of contraction does not increase and may in fact decrease (Note: that 1 μm is one millionth of a meter).

The Frank-Starling mechanism also allows the heart to adjust to changes in blood pressure. If systemic blood pressure is raised, the left ventricle has to generate higher pressure (and more force) to open the aortic valve. That workload -- which must be mounted to open the aortic valve, and is therefore impressed on the heart *after* it starts to contract -- is called *afterload*. (Note that afterload is essentially "pressure" work.) This increase in afterload may at first result in reducing the amount of blood pumped from the ventricle. This is turn leaves behind some blood that would have been ejected. The left-behind volume plus the volume from the next diastolic filling increases the next preload, and contractility again increases.

Although it would seem to be a good thing to dilate a ventricle by stretching the myofibrils, at least up to the point of not overextending the sarcomeres, there is a price to be paid. For the source of that price we look back to Pierre Simon, Marquis de Laplace, an 18th century polymath. Laplace demonstrated that the stress on the walls of a cylinder, in which there is a given pressure, is proportional to the cylinder's radius. Translated into our terms, a bigger ventricular cavity (which is somewhat cylindrical) means more tension on its walls at any given pressure. So it takes more energy -- that is, each myocyte has to work harder -- to squeeze a dilated ventricle than to squeeze a normal one.

Back to intrinsic control measures, one other is noteworthy. When the heart rate increases, the force of contraction also increases. This is because with increased heart rate there is a decrease in the time between beats and therefore less time for cytoplasmic $Ca^{2+}$ levels to fall after the action potential–induced increase. This results in increased intracellular $Ca^{2+}$ and increased contractility.

## OUTSIDERS

The really big changes in heart performance are mediated by the nervous system, or more specifically by the autonomic nervous system. As you may recall, this is the part of the nervous system that controls or modulates many basic functions that are not consciously controlled. Responding to internal stimuli, it helps to maintain a consistent internal environment; responding to external stimuli, it helps the body to meet changes and challenges in its external environment.

There are two arms of the autonomic nervous system: the sympathetic and the parasympathetic. Broadly speaking, the sympathetic system, which can discharge as a unit, promotes response to stress or risk -- the "fight or flight" reaction. The parasympathetic branch is more apt to act locally and discretely in an effort to conserve or restore energy. These two parts tend to work in a reciprocal fashion, with one down when the other is up. However, sympathetic and parasympathetic systems are not mirror images of one another. Some tissues are supplied with nerve fibers from only one or the other, and at times both systems may work together.

A brief review of nerve cells or neurons is in order. The cell body of the neuron houses the nucleus and organelles. Dendrites, usually short projections from the cell body, collect messages from the other neurons. The nerve fiber or axon is an elongated tubular extension of the neuron. It transmits its message to other nerve cells or to target cells. The propagated activity along an axon is an action potential or a series of action potentials.

A collection of cell bodies outside the central nervous system is called a ganglion, while a collection inside the central nervous system is referred to as a center or nucleus. Axons transmit their messages by releasing a neurotransmitter substance at their terminal ends. A synapse is the junction between two nerve cells across which a neurotransmitter passes.

The autonomic system has a basic two-neuron arrangement. The first neuron is in the central nervous system (CNS) and its axon is the preganglionic fiber. It synapses with the second neuron, which lies outside the CNS. The axon of this neuron is the postganglionic fiber. It extends to and communicates with cells in the target organ.

Parasympathetic fibers originate in the brain and brain stem. Neurons course from one of these areas to the heart via the vagus nerves. There they synapse with the second neuron in the pathway. These second neurons are short and their ganglia lie close to their target areas, the SA and AV nodes. This pattern is typical for a parasympathetic pathway -- long preganglionic fibers and short postganglionic fibers, with the latter lying near the target organ. The right vagus nerve affects the SA node chiefly and the left vagus affects the AV node chiefly.

When stimulated, these postganglionic fibers release the neurotransmitter acetylcholine. When the SA node is exposed to acetylcholine, the $K^+$ channels of its cells tend to stay open. The permeability to potassium increases, and the cell membrane hyperpolarizes. This sequence of events also opposes that gradual reduction in potassium permeability that contributes to spontaneous depolarization. Both of these factors slow spontaneous depolarization and this increases the time between heartbeats. In short, the heart rate goes down in response to parasympathetic activity.

In the AV node acetylcholine increases $K^+$ permeability and this hyperpolarizes the cell membranes. This slows conduction through the AV node by retarding excitation.

The sympathetic innervation of the heart is a more extensive system than the parasympathetic because it serves not just the SA and AV nodes but also the myocardial tissue. Here again we find the basic two-neuron units. The preganglionic fibers originate in the spinal cord where they can be affected by higher centers. They synapse with ganglia that lie in interconnecting chains, one on either side of the spinal column. The postganglionic fibers going to the heart from these ganglia are longer than their parasympathetic counterparts. They follow the large blood vessels and on reaching the heart form an extensive network across the epicardium. They then penetrate the myocardium, following the coronary vessel branches. When stimulated, these fibers release norepinephrine at their terminals.

The sympathetic system can effect a very big increase in cardiac output, both by increasing heart rate and by increasing the force of each contraction. (Cardiac output is the amount of blood pumped each minute, so it is determined by multiplying the heart rate times the stroke volume, the amount of blood pumped each beat.)

Norepinephrine released by the sympathetic fibers increases the permeability of the cells of the SA node to all three ions -- $Na^+$, $Ca^{2+}$, and $K^+$. However, the effect of the increased $Na^+$ and $Ca^{2+}$ currents exceeds that of the increased $K^+$ current, so the rate of spontaneous depolarization is increased, and heart rate increases. In addition, norepinephrine from sympathetic stimulation causes increased $Ca^{2+}$ to flow into myocytes through plasma membrane channels; this enhances the cells' contractility. Norepinephrine also promotes reuptake by the sarcoplasmic reticulum by stimulating its calcium pump; it does this by activating phospholamban. And norepinephrine inhibits binding of calcium to troponin. These last two effects increase the speed of relaxation. Thus the sympathetic system enhances both contraction and relaxation during the cardiac cycle. We will have an opportunity later to see how norepinephrine signals these activities.

This is a good place to reemphasize the fact that relaxation or diastole is more than simple myocardial elastic recoil. Sympathetic nervous system stimulation accelerates relaxation and increases filling.

These pathways, sympathetic and parasympathetic, can be stimulated or inhibited by various CNS centers. These in turn may be influenced by a number of sensing systems. These components -- a sensing system input synapsing with a control center output -- form reflex arcs.

One such sensing system is found in special receptors in the arch of the aorta and in the carotid arteries. These baroreceptors can sense sudden changes in blood pressure. If blood pressure is elevated, the baroreceptors sense this and relay that information to the parasympathetic and sympathetic systems. The former is stimulated and the latter is inhibited causing the heart rate to slow.

In addition there are stretch receptors in the atria that, when stimulated by increased atrial filling, effect an increase in heart rate. This reflex, also mediated by the autonomic system, is antagonistic to the baroreceptor reflex.

The autonomic system also responds to changes in arterial oxygen and carbon dioxide levels. The sensors of arterial oxygen and of carbon dioxide ($CO_2$) are located in the brain and also in the carotid arteries. Low oxygen and high carbon dioxide levels are triggers that can result in sympathetic stimulation.

Low oxygen in the blood perfusing the heart has direct effects as well. A modest reduction in coronary arterial oxygen level is stimulating, whereas a marked reduction is depressant. So, too, abnormal blood carbon dioxide can directly influence cardiac performance. Here, low $CO_2$ is stimulating and high $CO_2$ is depressant.

The adrenal gland medulla is one of the target organs of the sympathetic nervous system. When the sympathetic system is activated as a unit, the adrenal gland responds by releasing norepinephrine and also closely related epinephrine into the bloodstream. This second, humoral source of stimulant compounds greatly augments the sympathetic effect on the heart.

The heart has another, somewhat surprising, regulatory system. It can act as an endocrine organ by secreting a hormone called atrial natriuretic peptide (ANP). When the atrial walls are stretched, special cells there release ANP which causes the kidney to put out more urine -- that is, sodium and water. ANP also has some effect on blood vessel dilation. In this way the heart helps to regulate circulating blood volume and blood pressure.

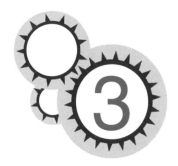

# THE ARTERIES

## REVIEW

How was that again?

The heart muscle cells -- which have inside them many little contractile units -- are linked together so that the whole heart tightens up in an orderly fashion on receiving the proper signal. The proper signal is a wave of electrical activity that sweeps over the heart, carried by a special conducting system over a specific pathway. It is initiated by special pacemaking cells. This signal results in a burst of calcium release into muscle cells' cytoplasm, triggering a shortening of the contrac-tile units. The sum of the contractions of all these units squeezes blood out of the heart in directions determined by internal valves, sending it in two different directions: to the lungs and to the general circulation. This is fol-lowed by relaxation and filling of the heart again. There is a host of mechanisms for varying the amount of blood pumped and for fine-tuning the whole performance. The heart is a star indeed.

What's next? Next we will talk about arteries. The heart may be reliable and hard working, but the arteries are really smart.

---

The role of the arteries is apt to look rather humble when compared to the heart's work. After all, the arteries merely deliver the blood to the capillaries. Granted, in doing so they reveal special design features that allow them to perform useful feats. Arteries are able to deliver blood with a smooth, nonfluctuating steady flow to the capillaries. They can do that largely because the arterial system is a pressure reservoir, providing a perpetual force to push blood into the capillaries.

The fact is, however, the arterial system does much more than just *deliver*. It is the smart part of the circulatory system; it is its brain trust. Small arteries *regulate* blood flow and *distribute* the precise amount of blood needed by a particular tissue or organ at any given time. The capillaries in the tissues and organs passively receive whatever their arteries present. Moreover, while delivering all these *various* amounts of blood, the arterial system maintains a *stable* pressure.

Let's see how the system works, and how it is able to reconcile its apparently divergent tasks.

## ON THE HYDRAULIC FILTER

What in their design allows the arteries to dampen out fluctuations in blood flow that the heart creates with its alternating systole and diastole? How do they turn pulsatile flow into steady flow?

The aorta and the other large arteries have distensible walls. These walls have abundant elastic fibers (elastin) arranged around their circumferences. This allows their diameters to be stretched. Recall that most of the heart's stroke volume is ejected into the arterial system during the early part of systole. During this time the amount of blood going into the arteries is greater than the amount coming out because the elastic arteries can bulge out. With the rest of systole and then diastole, little and then no blood enters the arteries but the elastic recoil of the distended arteries continues to push the blood downstream.

As the large arteries run to their target tissues and organs, they branch into smaller and smaller sizes, reaching the smallest, the arterioles. This reduction in diameter is marked. The aorta has a diameter of about 25 mm, while the average arteriolar diameter is around 0.03 mm. The small arteries and arterioles are the major *resistance* vessels in the circulatory system. It is here that resistance to flow is the greatest. Recall that in any system resistance increases markedly as the radius of its channel decreases. Indeed, resistance is inversely proportional to the fourth power of the radius, or

$$\text{Resistance} \propto \frac{1}{\text{Radius}^4}$$

This means that if a vessel's radius is halved its resistance goes up by a factor of 2 to the fourth power, or 16 times. Not only that, but the flow in that vessel would go down by a factor of 16 (Flow $\propto$ Radius$^4$). Note that a fall in blood pressure results from the increased resistance across the small arteries and the arterioles. The average pressure going in is 90 mm Hg and is 35 mm Hg coming out.

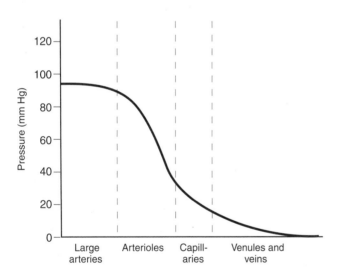

These high resistance small arteries and arterioles help create behind themselves a pressure head able to push blood steadily into the capillaries.

It is these two design features of the arteries -- elastic conduits and high-resistance end arteries -- that convert the heart's pulsatile output into steady flow by the time blood reaches the capillaries. This effect is called hydraulic filtering.

There is a practical benefit to hydraulic filtering, over and above the obvious one of providing a steady incoming flow for the capillaries. It improves the effi-

ciency of the heart. Tracing the reasons for that is an interesting exercise.

The heart would be more efficient if it produced continuous flow instead of intermittent flow. A simple reason is that an intermittent pump is not working -- is not creating flow -- a significant part of the time. That means when it is creating flow it has to catch up (pump more) during its active time to match the work of its continuously pumping counterpart.

To create a greater flow rate, any pump needs to use more force -- that is, to create more pressure (assuming resistance stays constant). Now work for a pump is really the product of pressure times volume moved. If we say volume moved in a given time for both kinds of pumps is the same, the pulsatile pump has had to create a greater pressure, if even for a short time, and has therefore had to work harder. It looks like this for the intermittent pump.

Shorter pumping time → ↑Flow rate

→ ↑Pressure → ↑Work

The distensibility (or, to the physiologist, the compliance) of the elastic arteries does two things that are really sides of the same coin. When distended, arteries store some of the energy of contraction which is then released to push blood downstream during the heart's off-time. In addition, the arterial ballooning reduces the pressure part of the equation, thus reducing the work.

The elastic arteries then team up with the heart to reduce some of the price the body pays for its choice of pulsatile over continuous pumping. If the arteries become stiffer, that price again rises.

## REGULATING AND DISTRIBUTING

Distribution of blood in the systemic circulation begins with large branches taking off from the largest artery, the aorta. These branches include arteries to the heart, head, limbs, gastrointestinal tract, kidneys, and pelvis. Here is the inflow part of the scheme of parallel circuits. (The outflow part is made up of veins draining these regions. These veins feed into the two largest veins, the superior and inferior venae cavae, which meet at the right atrium.)

Examining the anatomy of arteries, we see that form follows function. The essential functions required of arteries are that they (especially the large ones) be tough and elastic enough to handle the high and pulsatile pressure to which they are subjected and that they (especially the small ones) be able to vary their internal diameter size to allow more or less blood to flow through, while maintaining their role as high-resistance vessels.

Arteries have three layers. The innermost intima is a single layer of lining cells (the endothelium) and an underlying basement membrane. We will consider the roles of the endothelial cells in detail later. In medium-sized and large arteries a band of elastic fibers is found under the basement membrane. This is the internal elastic lamina. The middle layer or media has circumferentially arranged muscle cells that can alter the vessel circumference and enough elastic fibers and collagen (strong binding fibers) to withstand the pressure within. The outer layer, the adventitia, has longitudinally directed elastic fibers and collagen (for strength) as well as fibroblasts, macrophages, nerve fibers, and small blood vessels. (These last are the vasa vasorum, Latin for vessels' vessels.) As arteries get smaller the *proportion* of elastic fibers in the media decreases and the *proportion* of muscle cells increases. This makes sense because the small arteries participate in the resistance part of the hydraulic pump, not the compliance part. In the smallest arterioles the media consists of a single layer of muscle cells.

The kind of muscle cells found in the walls of arteries is smooth muscle. Here contractile elements are not lined up precisely, as they are in cardiac myocytes, so these cells do not exhibit bands or striations. Ar-

ranged around the circumference of the artery wall, they can cause the vessel to dilate when they relax and to constrict when they contract. Of course, dilatation is associated with an increase in blood flow and constriction with a decrease.

## VASCULAR SMOOTH MUSCLE CELLS -- HARMONIC TONES

The smart function of the circulatory system -- regulating and distributing blood essentially perfectly to the capillaries -- falls chiefly to the arterioles. The arterioles in turn rely on their smooth muscle cells. The smooth muscle cells are up to this responsibility because they have special talents. First, they can contract partially, not like striated muscle cells which are either in a contracting or relaxing phase. In fact, arterial smooth muscle cells are usually in a state of partial contraction. This condition of low level tension, referred to as tone, allows them to contract more (reducing blood flow) or to relax more (increasing blood flow). Arterial smooth muscle cells can maintain their tone with little energy expense even though they are exerting force. In addition, these cells can and do respond to a great variety of influences (as we will see) but they funnel these multiple influences to one basic regulatory pathway.

We begin with the contractile units of smooth muscle cells. As in cardiac muscle cell sarcomeres, actin and myosin are the key components and act as sliding filaments. Recall that in smooth muscle, contractile units are not lined up. They have no Z-lines but instead have

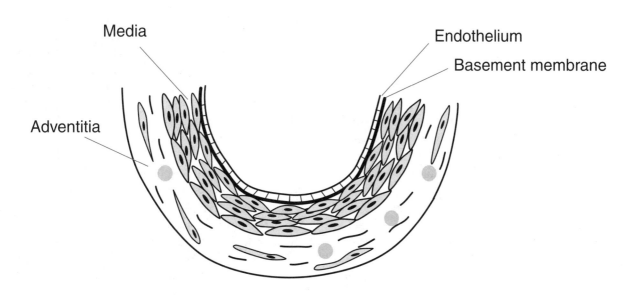

analogous structures called dense bodies to which actin filaments are anchored. There are more thin actin filaments in each contractile unit than are found in cardiac sarcomeres. (In smooth muscle cells there are 10 to 15 thin actin filaments to each thick myosin filament.) These contractile units form a diamond-shaped lattice within the cell. Their contraction results in the cell getting shorter and fatter. Dense bodies that are on the cell membrane may connect with the same structure on the adjacent cell, linking the cells' contraction activities. And like cardiac muscle cells, there are gap junctions between cells allowing for electrical communication.

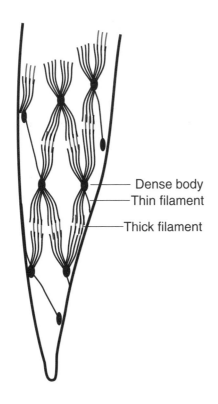

Dense body
Thin filament
Thick filament

Much of the special talent of smooth muscle cells derives from unique features of its crossbridging cycle. First of all, smooth muscle actin has no troponin. So to prepare for crossbridging there is no calcium ($Ca^{2+}$) binding to an actin component; instead, $Ca^{2+}$ acts indirectly by binding to the protein calmodulin (which is similar in structure to troponin). We already met calmodulin when we found it employed by cardiac myocytes to do another kind of work, activating the plasma membrane $Ca^{2+}$ pump.

This $Ca^{2+}$–calmodulin complex activates an enzyme, myosin kinase, that transfers a phosphate from adenosine triphosphate (ATP) onto the arm of *myosin*.

Only with this phosphate in place can the crossbridging cycle begin. (When it does begin, it proceeds much as it does in cardiac muscle cells, but with some important differences.)

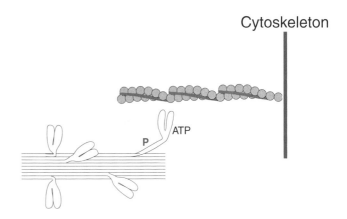

Cytoskeleton

P    ATP

So rising $Ca^{2+}$ in the cell cytoplasm results in more myosin being primed for crossbridging. Note however that this initial step (unlike the initial step in cardiac sarcomeres when $Ca^{2+}$ bonds to troponin on actin), has an energy cost of one ATP per myosin arm phosphorylated.

Crossbridge cycling continues until the $Ca^{2+}$ level falls. The rate of cycling is slower than it is in cardiac muscle sarcomeres but the force generated and the distance each unit shortens with each cycle are essentially the same. As the $Ca^{2+}$ level falls, $Ca^{2+}$–calmodulin falls and myosin kinase becomes inactive. Now the phosphate is removed from the myosin arm by another enzyme, myosin phosphatase.

So what's the big deal? This process is so far not a lot different from what we have seen before and it takes more energy. There is one detail of crossbridging, however, that has far-reaching consequences. When $Ca^{2+}$ falls, the myosin arm can have its phosphate removed (by myosin phosphatase) while it is attached to actin. If this occurs the attachment *remains* for an extended time. This allows the contractile unit and others like it in the smooth muscle cell (and therefore the cell itself) to sustain partial contraction, or tone, for a time and to do it with little energy expended because ATP is not being continually consumed. This prolonged attachment is called the latch phenomenon. Even though there was additional energy expense at first, overall this latch phenomenon reduces the energy cost to 1/300th the amount of ATP that striated muscle would need to sustain the same force.

As a result of being able to latch, smooth muscle

cells have a set of crossbridge states not available to cardiac muscle cells. In cardiac muscle cells, when $Ca^{2+}$ concentration is up, the binding sites on actin for myosin heads are available and crossbridges form, cycle, and continue to cycle. Sarcomeres progressively shorten. The cardiac myocyte contracts. When $Ca^{2+}$ falls, the binding sites on actin are no longer available to myosin heads for attachment. Thus, binding stops. The sarcomeres lengthen. The cardiac myocyte relaxes.

Compare that to smooth muscle cells. Here also $Ca^{2+}$ is the regulator. When $Ca^{2+}$ is up, the myosin arm is phosphorylated, allowing crossbridges to form, cycle, and continue to cycle. The contractile units shorten. The smooth muscle cell contracts. When $Ca^{2+}$ falls, the myosin arm is dephosphorylated. No new attachments of myosin heads to actin occur. But those *already* established proceed through the cycle at a slowed rate. The attachment lingers. (These states of cycling in the face of fallen $Ca^{2+}$ level cannot occur in cardiac cells.) The effect is the sum of multiple crossbridge cycle states with many attachments lingering in multiple contractile units. This can produce partial smooth muscle cell contraction -- no progressive contraction and no relaxation -- at least for a time. If the $Ca^{2+}$ stays down (or falls lower), detachments ultimately occur and the contractile units lengthen. The smooth muscle cell relaxes.

The $Ca^{2+}$ level in the smooth muscle cell determines its contractile state. Here that state is not off or on, contracted or relaxed. Instead it may be somewhere in between, in a whole range of modulations or gradations. Altering the $Ca^{2+}$ level is the way to get to the smooth muscle cell. This is the basic regulatory pathway alluded to earlier.

Let's first look at the ways by which calcium in the smooth muscle cell can be varied. Then we will consider how agents that influence the cell use those means of changing intracellular calcium.

## UPS AND DOWNS OF CALCIUM

Calcium can enter the smooth muscle cell from outside through the plasma membrane and it can be released into the cytoplasm from stores in the sarcoplasmic reticulum. There are two ways $Ca^{2+}$ can pass in through the plasma membrane. A change in the membrane potential can open voltage-regulated $Ca^{2+}$ channels. $Ca^{2+}$ enters, eliciting contraction (*electromechanical coupling*). Other plasma membrane calcium channels open in response to a specific chemical mediator, a process of *pharmacomechanical coupling*. $Ca^{2+}$ from the smooth muscle sarcoplasmic reticulum is released only by the means of pharmacomechanical coupling. $Ca^{2+}$ is removed from smooth muscle cell cytoplasm by being pumped back out through the plasma membrane or back into the sarcoplasmic reticulum; or it is traded for sodium via the plasma membrane exchanger.

Electromechanical coupling, as noted, depends on voltage-regulated $Ca^{2+}$ channels. The resting membrane potential across smooth muscle cell plasma membrane is usually $-48$ mV. This is largely an expression of the membrane's potassium permeability but with a bit more contribution from $Ca^{2+}$ permeability than we saw in cardiac myocytes. Thus, the membrane potential is less negative in vascular smooth muscle cells than it is in cardiac myocytes. If the membrane potential is made less negative (that is, depolarized) more voltage-regulated $Ca^{2+}$ channels open and $Ca^{2+}$ enters the cell. This results in greater smooth muscle contraction, vasoconstriction, and reduced flow. Conversely, if the membrane potential is made more negative (hyperpolarized) more of the $Ca^{2+}$ channels close, and the $Ca^{2+}$ level in the cell falls ($Ca^{2+}$ having been removed by pump or exchange). This results in smooth muscle cell relaxation (or less contraction), vasodilatation, and increased flow. Restated, depolarization causes vasoconstriction and hyperpolarization causes vasodilatation.

This electromechanical coupling can be very sensitive. The change in membrane potential does not require an action potential with its spike of depolarization. Just a slight change in potassium ($K^+$) permeance can make a difference. How slight and what difference?

There are around 50,000 $K^+$ channels in each smooth muscle cell's plasma membrane. If an additional three of these open, the membrane potential goes from $-48$ mV to $-50$ mV. This bit of hyperpolarization can close enough $Ca^{2+}$ channels (again, voltage regulated) to effect a decrease in the intracellular $Ca^{2+}$ level. (One open $Ca^{2+}$ channel of this type can let 1.4 million ions into the cell each second, so one closed channel keeps that many out.)

This reduction in $Ca^{2+}$ can decrease vascular tone. We know that even a small amount of relaxation, leading to a greater vessel circumference, increases blood flow. How amazing that opening these few additional potassium channels in each vascular smooth muscle cell can cause, through a series of amplifying events, increased flow in an arteriole.

Action potentials can and do occur in vascular smooth muscle cells, though they are blunted affairs with no overshoot and with minimal spread. Smooth muscle cells do not have fast sodium channels, so the change in membrane potential during an action potential is chiefly due to a rapid increase in $Ca^{2+}$ permeance.

Because action potentials do not play such a primary role in smooth muscle as they do in cardiac muscle, smooth muscle cells have no need for T-tubules to transmit an action potential deep inside. Indeed they do not have T-tubules but instead have small shallow sacs in the plasma membrane (caveoli).

Intracellular $Ca^{2+}$, in the vascular smooth muscle cell, can also be affected by pharmacologic means (pharmacomechanical coupling) and this usually occurs without altering the membrane potential. The agent can be a neurotransmitter, almost always from a sympathetic nerve ending. A molecular agent can also reach the smooth muscle cell from the blood or from other cells in the neighborhood. So depending on how it is delivered, an influence can be neural or humoral.

The particular agent is called an agonist (from the Greek word αγωνιστησ, which means "one who contends for a prize"), or a ligand because it binds to a particular agent. This fitting of an agonist to its receptor on a smooth muscle cell membrane elicits a special response. Because we are focusing on pharmacomechanical coupling, the responses we are interested in are those in $Ca^{2+}$ channels in the plasma membrane and those in the sarcoplasmic reticulum that affect $Ca^{2+}$ release from there. Note what a different role the sarcoplasmic reticulum plays in smooth muscle cells compared to cardiac muscle cells. It does not release a burst of $Ca^{2+}$ but rather responds in a measured fashion to a measured stimulus.

## G WHIZZES

Pharmacomechanical coupling has some problems. Unlike its counterpart it does not have an array of calcium channels eager to respond to a relatively simple environment change (specifically, a change in membrane potential). An agonist somehow has to tell each of its targeted calcium channels what to do. Those channels may not be only on the cell (on the plasma membrane) but may be in the cell (in the sarcoplasmic reticulum). Furthermore, the body is likely to want to modulate the agonist's effect. Pharmacomechanical coupling solves these problems by using a system of signaling, which the body also uses with great frequency and great success elsewhere. This system is G protein signaling and it is well worth looking at. Investigation of this system has so far won three Nobel prizes for different research groups and there could be more in the future as these processes are so fundamental to cell functioning and interaction.

G proteins are guanine nucleotide-binding proteins (guanine is, of course, a close relative of adenine of ATP). This family of proteins relays signals from each of more than 1000 different membrane receptors to many different intracellular targets, including ion channels and enzymes. (There are, of course, many other membrane receptors which use different signaling devices.) The basic scheme starts with an agonist binding to its specific receptor on the cell membrane. The G protein lying just under the plasma membrane is bound to this receptor that straddles the membrane with a piece sticking outside to receive the agonist and a piece sticking inside.

The G protein has three parts: alpha, beta, gamma. When inactive, the alpha piece is bound to guanosine diphosphate (GDP) and the alpha-GDP is in turn bound to beta and gamma, which stay together. When the agonist, combining with the outside part of the receptor, activates this system, GDP is released and guanosine triphosphate (GTP) binds to alpha. Now the alpha-GTP piece comes apart from the beta-gamma piece and both (alpha-GTP and beta-gamma) separate from the receptor. Each part is now free in the cell to activate a specific target or set of targets.

As is so often the case, nature takes this basic plan and, by varying its parts, creates a large number of different combinations, each acting as a separate signal. To wit, there are 16 alphas, 6 betas, and 12 gammas. Each alpha type (with its GTP) and each beta-gamma type can have either a different target or a different effect on a common target. (These targets, incidentally, are called *effectors* because they are acted on to produce an effect.)

The activity of the signal stops when the GTP hooked to alpha is hydrolyzed to GDP. The alpha-GDP piece is now inactive and it binds to beta-gamma, turning that piece off as well. The total group rejoins the receptor. Note that by facilitating the hydrolysis of GTP, the cell can shorten and weaken the signal; and by inhibiting the hydrolysis it can lengthen and strengthen the signal.

It all looks like this:

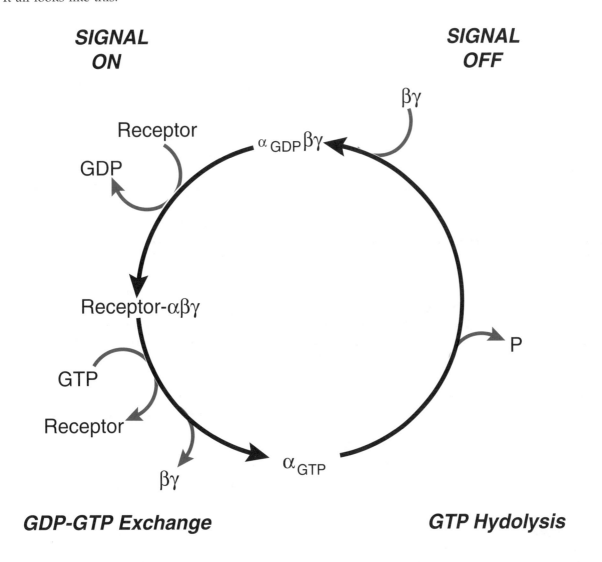

**SIGNAL ON**

**SIGNAL OFF**

Receptor

GDP

$\alpha_{GDP}\beta\gamma$

$\beta\gamma$

Receptor-$\alpha\beta\gamma$

GTP

Receptor

$\beta\gamma$

$\alpha_{GTP}$

P

**GDP-GTP Exchange**

**GTP Hydolysis**

## AGENTS OF CHANGE

Now let's get back to arterial and arteriolar smooth muscle cells and see what it is they respond to that allows their vessels to make proper distribution of blood to the body. Now we can also distinguish by what means these numerous influences cause their responses.

Proper distribution of blood is the result of increasing flow here, decreasing it there, always taking into account local tissue needs under various conditions and overall systemic needs under various conditions. At any given time all needs are important and yet some are more important than others. For example, circulation to the heart and brain must be ensured at all times; muscles need more blood during exercise; when it's hot, the skin needs more blood to be routed to it to dissipate heat. This is all done with virtual perfection. Clearly some influences need to have widespread effects, whereas others must be directed to a narrow niche.

## *ARTERIOLE, REGULATE THYSELF*

There are local or intrinsic controls of blood flow. There are also extrinsic controls from outside the tissues. Intrinsic controls often allow specific tissues or organs to act in their own behalf to *increase or decrease* blood flow when necessary. They also can help *maintain* blood flow, stabilizing it within a required range. We have noted the need to vary blood flow but it is also important to maintain a steady blood supply to tissues and to avoid excessive "peaks and valleys." This stabilizing kind of intrinsic control is commonly called autoregulation.

There are two chief mechanisms for autoregulation. One is the myogenic mechanism. Here vascular smooth muscle *contracts* in response to an increase in pressure on the vessel wall and relaxes when there is a decrease in wall pressure. There are stretch-activated sodium and calcium channels in the arteriolar wall which when stretched tend to open and thereby induce depolarization. This opens voltage regulated $Ca^{2+}$ channels leading to increased intracellular $Ca^{2+}$ and vasoconstriction. In this way an increase in blood flow caused by an abrupt increase in pressure is returned to previous flow rate by vascular smooth muscle contraction and vessel narrowing.

A second scheme is flow-dependent dilation. Here an increase in flow in an arteriole effects vessel *relaxation*. This occurs because stress exerted by the streaming blood on the vessel wall triggers a cascade of events that results in reducing vessel smooth muscle intracellular $Ca^{2+}$. These events depend on another very important signaling system (another Nobel-prize-winning elucidation). Here the active factor is nitric oxide (NO). Before the identity of nitric oxide was established it was called endothelium-derived relaxing factor (EDRF). The fact that EDRF turned out to be this simple molecule was quite unexpected. Even more surprising has been the enormous variety of biologic appearances NO makes. It is involved in smooth muscle tone, neural signaling, immune function, and blood clotting -- and this list is incomplete.

For our discussion we will focus on how NO effects arteriolar smooth muscle relaxation. When an endothelial cell in an arteriole is subjected to an increase in shear stress from increased flow, $Ca^{2+}$ influx occurs. (Recall that shear stress is the frictional drag from moving blood, in this case on the endothelial cell membrane.) This $Ca^{2+}$, in the *endothelial* cell, combines with a familiar protein, calmodulin. The $Ca^{2+}$–calmodulin complex activates the enzyme NO synthase which converts L-arginine and oxygen into L-citrulline and NO. The NO quickly diffuses into the smooth muscle cell below. There it catalyzes the conversion of guanosine triphosphate to cyclic guanosine monophosphate (cGMP). The cGMP activates a large number of phosphorylating enzymes (kinases), which do a great

number of things, all of which tend to lower $Ca^{2+}$ in the smooth muscle cell. The cGMP, through the actions of these enzymes, causes an increase in $Ca^{2+}$ extrusion by stimulating the plasma membrane $Ca^{2+}$ pump and the $Na^+$–$Ca^{2+}$ exchanger. It causes increased activity of the sarcoplasmic reticulum $Ca^{2+}$ pump. It downregulates $Ca^{2+}$ channels, voltage regulated and agonist responsive. And it interferes with $Ca^{2+}$ release from the sarcoplasmic reticulum.

These two mechanisms of autoregulation tend to offset each other. If there is an increase in arteriolar pressure with associated increase in flow, the myogenic mechanism will promote vasoconstriction and the flow-dependent dilation will promote vasodilatation. The end result will be played out as a kind of arteriolar yin and yang.

On the other hand, if some additional factor such as enhanced tissue metabolic activity causes arteriolar dilatation then the myogenic mechanism and flow-dependent dilation both act to support increased flow.

Tissue metabolic activity has a great effect on local blood flow. When metabolic activity increases in a tissue a lot of things happen there, not only in the cells, but also in the interstitial fluid which bathes the cells. Oxygen level goes down (from increased use), carbon dioxide goes up (lowering the pH), potassium is released by the active cells into the interstitial fluid, interstitial fluid osmolality (total particle concentration) goes up, and some specific compounds, like adenosine and prostacyclin, may be produced. Probably all of these events contribute to increasing local tissue blood flow.

Reduction of oxygen may act in several ways, including promoting NO formation and sensitizing vascular smooth muscle cells to hyperpolarizing influences. An increase in extracellular $H^+$ (caused by raising $CO_2$ in the tissues) also contributes to hyperpolarizing the cell membrane. Increased potassium in interstitial fluid may have a hyperpolarizing effect as it stimulates the cells' sodium pump.

A number of metabolically active tissues produce adenosine. It diffuses to the vascular smooth muscle cells where its membrane receptor is G protein coupled. Here again the ultimate effect is to hyperpolarize the cell membrane.

Prostacyclin is produced by endothelial cells. It also activates a G protein coupled receptor on the smooth muscle cell. The result is an increase in a compound called cyclic adenosine monophosphate (cAMP) in the cell, which in this case leads to closing $Ca^{2+}$ channels and vasodilatation. (More on cAMP later.)

## RECEIVING ORDERS

Extrinsic control of blood flow through arteries is both neural (via the autonomic, and chiefly sympathetic, nervous system) and humoral (via the bloodstream). The neural controls may be widely applied, as in a generalized sympathetic discharge, or may be directed to a local area. Parasympathetic stimulation is usually focally targeted. A humoral agonist that is blood borne is, of course, widely distributed.

Sympathetic neural stimulation is ongoing with greater or lesser activity to produce more or less tone or vasoconstriction. The directing neurons originate in the central nervous system medulla where there are pressor centers that promote output over the sympathetic system, and depressor centers that inhibit output from the sympathetic centers. At the ends of the second sympathetic neurons (in this case, in the artery walls) the neurotransmitter released is norepinephrine. We have already seen that norepinephrine has a number of cardiac effects but we left details of how it works inside cells until now.

There are two basic categories of receptors for norepinephrine, alpha and beta. (These receptors are often referred to as adrenergic, meaning "stimulated by an adrenal hormone.") These were initially distinguished because they have differing agonist affinities, are blocked by different agents, and at times have different actions when coupled with agonists. As these were investigated more closely, subgroups of both alpha and beta receptors were found. As it turns out, these are all G protein coupled receptors.

The proportion of alpha and beta receptors is different in different blood vessels. Both are usually present. The alpha receptors in blood vessels that we are most interested in are those designated alpha-1. When norepinephrine, released by a sympathetic nerve ending, binds to an alpha-1 adrenergic receptor, the G protein signal activates its effector, the enzyme phospholipase C. This enzyme cleaves a special membrane phospholipid (this one is a complex molecule with fatty acids and a phosphorylated ring structure all hooked onto glycerol). The products are important, but especially important is inositol 1,4,5 triphosphate (IP3), the

ring structure with three phosphates. IP3 is a messenger that causes release of $Ca^{2+}$ from the sarcoplasmic reticulum. This, of course, promotes smooth muscle contraction and vasoconstriction.

The beta adrenergic receptor in blood vessels is designated beta-2. It responds preferentially to epinephrine circulating in the blood (a circulating humoral agent, not a neural agent).

Epinephrine and norepinephrine are structurally very closely related and are both classed as catecholamines. The chief source of epinephrine is the adrenal gland. When epinephrine couples with a beta-2 receptor it promotes vasodilatation.

How does this happen? The G protein signals an effector called adenylyl cyclase. This enzyme catalyzes the production of cAMP. The cAMP activates a protein kinase, which in turn phosphorylates (and thereby activates) a number of other enzymes. These promote lowering of intracellular $Ca^{2+}$ and consequently effect vasodilatation. They inhibit calcium channel opening; promote potassium channel opening (causing hyperpolarization); stimulate the sodium/calcium exchange; and inhibit release of IP3. They even go a step beyond affecting the $Ca^{2+}$ level in the cell, and reduce the activity of myosin kinase.

Two things about these beta-2 receptors are noteworthy. Despite all the activity they can stir up through cAMP, alpha activity can overcome their affect. Beta-2 receptors can also be quickly downregulated (desensitized) if stimulated over time.

Now that we know about G protein signaling, we need to go back and pick up some old business: how beta receptors in the heart cause responses when stimulated. Beta-1 receptors in the heart couple with norepinephrine. In cardiac muscle cells norepinephrine stimulates adenylyl cyclase (via a G protein signal, of course) to produce cAMP. Here, however, the activated protein kinase acts on enzymes that promote opening of $Ca^{2+}$ channels. This augments $Ca^{2+}$ influx into the cell and facilitates cardiac muscle cell contraction. In the cells with pacemaking capability, this same mechanism leads to increased opening not only of $Ca^{2+}$ channels but also of $K^+$ and $Na^+$ channels.

The parasympathetic nervous system innervation of blood vessels is much less than the sympathetic. But there are some vessels that receive parasympathetic nerve fibers. These include some vessels in the gastrointestinal tract and vessels in the genitalia and urinary bladder. These vessels all together represent only a small proportion of the body's "resistance vessels." As you recall, the agonist released by parasympathetic second neurons is acetylcholine. When acetylcholine couples with its receptor (a "cholinergic" receptor), the G protein signals lead to reduction of IP3 production and can also inhibit adenylyl cyclase, thus reducing cAMP which in this case lowers intracellular $Ca^{2+}$. Acetylcholine can also act on endothelial cells to induce production of NO, causing vasodilatation.

Let's look at one last piece of old business. Acetylcholine has an interesting effect on the heart's sinoatrial and atrioventricular nodes. Stimulation of its receptor opens $K^+$ channels, causing hyperpolarization. Here the G protein signals without intermediate steps and the beta-gamma piece acts *directly* on the $K^+$ channels.

Note again that the body can take one multistage pathway and tailor it to achieve different ends. We have seen a G protein signal that increases cAMP to lower intracellular $Ca^{2+}$; another that increases cAMP to raise $Ca^{2+}$; and still another that lowers cAMP to lower $Ca^{2+}$. We have seen catecholamines use G protein signaling and acetylcholine use G protein signaling. We have seen alpha-GTP piece activity and beta-gamma piece activity. Finally you have probably already guessed that a cell can vary the level of cAMP activity by influencing its breakdown. The enzyme phosphodiesterase, which hydrolyzes cAMP, can be increased or decreased in a variety of ways.

## Humors

Epinephrine is the leading humoral influence on circulation. It is secreted into the bloodstream by the adrenal gland's medulla. Epinephrine acts on all adrenergic receptors and is the agonist preferred by beta-2 receptors.

There are a number of other substances that circulate in the blood that act on resistance vessels and thereby affect blood pressure. The most potent vasoconstrictor produced by the body is angiotensin. It has an interesting lineage. Renin, an enzyme made in the kidney, is released when baroreceptors there sense a fall in blood pressure and when there is an increase in sympathetic nerve activity. (It is also secreted when special kidney cells sense a fall in sodium chloride in the blood.) Renin cleaves angiotensinogen (a circulating protein made by the liver) to form angiotensin I. This then is

converted to angiotensin II by angiotensin-converting enzyme (ACE) on the surface of endothelial cells. Angiotensin I (or just angiotensin) acts by promoting release of IP3 in vascular smooth muscle cells (yes, another G protein signal is involved). Angiotensin also directly stimulates the pressor center in the central nervous system (CNS); and it stimulates release of epinephrine from the adrenal medulla. Lastly, angiotensin augments norepinephrine release from sympathetic nerve terminals. Note the positive feedback loop. Sympathetic activity, via the neurotransmitter norepinephrine, induces renin output. This leads to angiotensin formation, which increases norepinephrine release.

Angiotensin also has an indirect way of raising blood pressure. It stimulates the adrenal gland cortex to secrete the hormone aldosterone. Aldosterone acts on the kidney to promote conservation of sodium and water and thereby increases circulating volume.

Endothelin is another vasoconstrictor. It is made, obviously, by endothelial cells. It acts on nearby smooth muscle cells but is also released into the bloodstream.

## Reflexes -- Overarc(h)ing Principles

Reflexes carried by the autonomic nervous system are part of the extrinsic controls of circulation, and are especially active in influencing blood pressure. In the short term, the most important stabilizers of blood pressure are the arterial baroreceptors. You recall them from their effect on cardiac activity; indeed, these are the same receptors found in the carotid arteries and in the arch of the aorta. The activity of this reflex arc serves once again to emphasize that maintaining blood pressure is done in large part by varying the resistance in the small arteries and arterioles; this is done by modulating the amount of sympathetic activity emanating from the CNS medulla. When the baroreceptors sense higher blood pressure (when they "feel" the increase in stretch and deformation caused by an increase in blood pressure) they send more neural messages to the appropriate place in the medulla. This *inhibits* outgoing sympathetic nerve impulses, thus reducing norepinephrine release at the ends of these nerve fibers in vessel walls and causing blood pressure to fall. You will recall the effects this sympathetic inhibition has on the heart -- lowering heart rate and contractility, and thereby lowering cardiac output.

Conversely, a fall in blood pressure causes less

input from the baroreceptors. This releases the center in the CNS medulla to increase the sympathetic nerve activity.

The atria also contain baroreceptors. These have quite complex activities. Among their responses to tension and stretching is a reflex-mediated reduction in sympathetic discharge from the CNS medulla to blood vessels. In addition, these baroreceptors, when stimulated, can initiate a reflex that reduces renin release (and consequently reduces angiotensin and aldosterone), and can reduce the release of the peptide vasopressin from the pituitary.

Vasopressin, despite its name, has little or no activity on vascular smooth muscle cells in its usual blood level range. It does influence the kidneys to conserve and retain water. (The other name for vasopressin is antidiuretic hormone.) So increased neural activity from baroreceptors (this includes the arterial ones) gets passed along from the CNS medulla to the midbrain and beyond to the posterior pituitary, which responds by reducing vasopressin output. The kidneys then excrete more water, with a resulting fall in vascular volume. It looks like this:

Increase in arterial stretch (higher pressure or higher volume)
→ Message to CNS medulla
→ Message to pituitary
→ Decreased release vasopressin (ADH)
→ Kidney excretes more water
→ Lower vascular volume and lower blood pressure

Of course, if baroreceptor stimulation is reduced, the scheme works the other way, resulting in an increase in vascular volume.

Recall that there are also a number of chemoreceptors in the body that can affect sympathetic activity. CNS as well as aortic and carotid chemoreceptors are sensitive to changes in oxygen, carbon dioxide, and pH levels. A fall in blood oxygen and a rise in blood carbon dioxide (with a fall in pH) result in vasoconstriction.

I have alluded to vasopressin and aldosterone and their effect on vascular volume. This only hinted at an important fact: the volume of fluid in the circulatory system helps determine blood pressure.

Responsibility for long-term blood pressure control (here we are talking in terms of days and weeks) falls largely to the kidneys. They respond to a number of factors. For it is the kidneys, reacting to such factors

as blood flow, blood composition, aldosterone, vasopressin (ADH), and atrial naturetic peptide, that determine the volume of blood that circulates. Once again, blood volume is a major determinant of blood pressure.

## WHAT IS THIS THING CALLED BLOOD PRESSURE?

Imagine if the only way to check someone's blood pressure would be the direct method of sticking a needle into a large artery and connecting the needle to a measuring device. In reality, measuring blood pressure is a simple procedure. This is good, because blood pressure is important and it can be measured frequently if need be.

We use an indirect but valid method, employing a sphygmomanometer (*sphygmo* meaning pulse; *manometer* meaning a pressure gauge). This is the familiar cuff with an inflatable bag inside. The cuff is attached to a manometer, often a mercury (Hg) column. The pressure in the air bag is transmitted to the mercury column.

Blood pressure is usually measured in the upper arm because it is easily accessible and the artery is large enough to reflect very closely the pressure in the aorta. (There is not enough resistance in the system at this level to have caused a significant pressure drop between the aorta and the brachial artery.) The cuff is wrapped around the arm and inflated to a pressure above the systolic blood pressure. This pressure is transmitted to the arm, and blood flow through the brachial artery is occluded. No blood now flows to that part of this artery which lies under the crease of the elbow. The measurer listens over this area with a stethoscope, and gradually lowers the cuff pressure by slightly opening a valve. The pressure exerted on the arm by the cuff is in turn gradually lowered. At a level just below the systolic blood pressure, a small amount of blood escapes through the artery, flowing downstream where the measurer is listening. She hears a sound. That sound is produced by the impact of that spurt of blood as it hits the static blood in the artery under the stethoscope. The pressure shown on the manometer at that moment is the systolic blood pressure. The measurer continues to lower the cuff pressure until the sound goes away. That pressure -- also shown on the manometer -- is the diastolic blood pressure, for it is at that point that flow in the artery is again continuous.

So when you hear that your blood pressure is

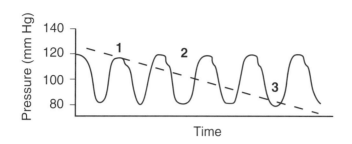

1. Sound first heard
2. Sound audible
3. Sound goes away

120/80 (which is the standard normal pressure at rest), it means that 120 mm Hg is your highest arterial pressure during systole and that 80 mm Hg is your lowest arterial pressure during diastole. The average arterial pressure during one cardiac cycle is the *mean arterial pressure.* Normal is 90 mm Hg. Mean arterial pressure depends on the two factors, cardiac output and peripheral resistance.

Pulse pressure, the difference between systolic and diastolic arterial pressures, is an interesting derivative. Obviously, it is usually about 40 mm Hg. Pulse pressure is determined by stroke volume and by arterial compliance (or distensibility). Why is that? Stretching the arterial system with a spurt of blood raises the pressure there: the bigger the spurt, the greater is the rise.

Additionally, the harder it is to stretch the arteries, the greater the rise. So increasing stroke volume or decreasing arterial compliance raises pulse pressure.

Finally, we come to what is perhaps the most familiar thing about arteries, the pulse -- that thrust we can feel over an artery. The pulse is really a pressure wave that is initiated by the ejection of blood during systole into the aorta. It travels faster than the blood itself and its velocity varies inversely with arterial compliance. Thus, the pulse velocity and the pulse pressure are higher in some of the smaller stiffer arteries than they are in the larger, more elastic ones. Of course, at some point the arteries are so small that first their mean pressure falls and then their pulse is dampened out.

# THE CAPILLARIES

## REVIEW

That was pretty hard. What is the short version?

The arteries receive blood from the heart and distribute it to the capillaries. In so doing, the arterial system, with its elastic conduit vessels and high-resistance end vessels, acts as a hydraulic filter, dampening fluctuations in flow while maintaining a pressure reservoir. Regulating the distribution of blood to capillaries is largely the responsibility of small arteries and arterioles. The smooth muscle in the walls of these vessels is maintained in a state of partial contraction that can increase or decrease to alter vessel diameter. This in turn alters flow through the vessel to the passively receiving capillaries. The tone of smooth muscle of the small arteries and arterioles is determined chiefly by the calcium level inside smooth muscle cells. That tone varies in response to a large number of influences -- autoregulation mechanisms, tissue metabolic activity, and extrinsic agents, both neural and hormonal. Teaming up with the kidneys, which regulate blood volume, this cleverly balanced system is able to maintain a steady pressure reservoir and at the same time is able to meet the blood flow needs of all the tissues and organs.

Are capillaries next? Yes, capillaries and endothelial cells, where most of the action is.

We have extolled the heart for its mechanical correctness and for its power. We have lauded the arterial system for its regulatory cleverness. Now what can we say about capillaries? We can say that capillaries are the reason the circulatory system exists. They deliver what the cells of the body need and pick up what they do not. We can say that the endothelial cells, which alone form capillaries, are the true heroes. They are astoundingly gifted and versatile. We are just now beginning to appreciate many of the talents of endothelial cells.

### STRENGTH IN NUMBERS

Capillaries are made up of a single layer of endothelial cells. Their walls are very thin (0.5–1.0 μm) and their average diameter only about the size of a red blood cell (7–8 μm). There many capillaries -- as many as 40 billion -- in the body. This accomplishes a most important goal: no cell is farther than 0.1 mm from a capillary.

Capillaries form networks of basically parallel connections between arterioles and venules (small veins). Their average length is 1 mm.

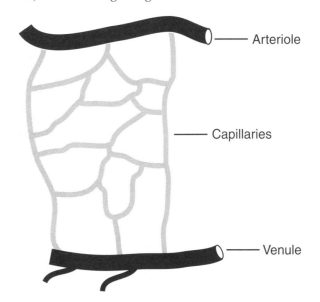

Arteriole

Capillaries

Venule

The total surface area of capillaries is huge (600 m²) and yet only about 5% of the blood volume (250 mL out of 5 liters) is in the capillary system at any given time. By this design, the relatively small volume of blood that occupies the capillary system is exposed to a very large surface area.

Flow through capillaries is relatively slow. Of course, this part of the circulatory system has to accept and pass along the same volume of blood (5 liters each minute at rest) that the heart pumps; but the velocity of flow in each capillary segment is less than that in the arterial or venous system. This is because the total area of all the cross sections of capillaries is so large: 6000 cm². (Compare this to the aorta with its 4.5 cm² cross sectional area.) It is like a river flowing into a lake and then narrowing into a river again. The same amount of water is flowing into and out from the lake, but the velocity of flow in the lake itself is much slower than in the river. We can calculate the average velocity of blood flow through the capillaries -- about 1 mm/sec; however, this number is not very meaningful because the flow rate is so variable. That is because at any given time, within the network of parallel connections, some capillaries will be receiving blood and some will not. In a perfect parallel arrangement with capillaries of equal size and length this would not be true, of course. Each capillary would get an equal share of whatever flow the feeding arteriole brings. But note from the picture that the arrangement of capillaries, while basically in parallel, is quite varied and forms a tortuous network. These tiny vessels also have a range of maximum diameters. Thus, an arteriole that is not fully dilated will establish circulation through some but not all the paths of this network.

One way the body has of increasing oxygen supply to cells (like active skeletal muscle cells) is to perfuse, or "open up," more capillaries, as the arterioles dilate. This reduces the distance oxygen has to diffuse to reach many cells' mitochondria. In skeletal muscle cells only about one-third of the capillaries carry blood during resting conditions. During strenuous exercise, however, they are all perfused, so the delivery of oxygen to those mitochondria is much quicker. Remember, diffusion time is proportional not to the distance a molecule travels but to the square of that distance.

One apparent inconsistency merits note. When we talked about the arterial system we said that arterioles were the high-resistance part of the circulatory system because they have such small diameters. Yet here we see capillaries with still smaller diameters. There are so many capillaries arranged in multiple, basically parallel circuits and the total cross sectional area of capillaries is so large that the resistance offered by the capillary system is relatively small.

Changes in capillary diameter are passive, reflecting what is happening with the arterioles and venules. For example, if the precapillary arteriole is dilated and the postcapillary venule is narrowed, the capillary clearly will be distended. So the question arises: even if the pressure in capillaries is relatively small (averaging 26 mm Hg), why are these very thin-walled vessels not blown out? It turns out that tension on a vessel wall is proportional to not only the pressure but also to the radius of the vessel (Laplace again). Because the radius of a capillary is so small, there is little wall tension. Consider as a comparison the aorta with its much larger radius: even though its pressure is only three to four times that in the capillaries, its wall tension is 12,000 times greater.

## FAIR EXCHANGES

The exchange that occurs across the capillary, the delivery and pickup, is really the movement of materials between the capillary and the fluid that bathes the cells, the interstitial fluid. This is the result of three processes -- diffusion, filtration, and pinocytosis (literally "cell drinking," a special packaging technique most cells have). Diffusion is the most important of these three and is a passive process. Diffusion in and out of a capillary depends on the concentration gradient of the diffusing substance, the permeability of the capillary to that substance, and capillary surface area. Permeability is enhanced by the presence of pores between endothelial cells. Many small molecules such as water, $Na^+$, $Cl^-$, and glucose readily go through these pores; larger molecules, over a molecular weight of 60,000, cannot pass. Lipid-soluble molecules can go through the endothelial cells. Oxygen and carbon dioxide use both routes. The diffusion of most small molecules is usually completed in the very beginning part of the capillary.

Some tissues prefer easier access to what is in the capillaries, and some less access. Variations in the basic capillary structure help accommodate those preferences. *Fenestrated endothelium* has small round, window-like bare areas exposing the basement membrane. As a result water, ions, and small molecules (but not proteins) get through more readily than in the standard model. Sometimes the endothelium is even *discontinuous*, having open areas in which the basement membrane is absent. This allows even many proteins to get through.

On the other extreme, some tissues require *tight endothelial junctions* with no pores, windows, or breaks so that everything going in and out of the capillaries has to go through an endothelial cell.

Before we get to the process of capillary filtration we must backtrack. When I discussed movement of molecules across membranes (see Chapter 2), I left something out. You may have wondered about it at the time. I dealt only with the movement of those molecules dissolved in water (the solute) and *not* with the movement of the water itself (the solvent). Water also may pass through semipermeable membranes and it goes toward greater solute concentration. This flow is called *osmosis*. Note that the higher the concentration of solute in a solution, the lower is the "concentration" of water. Osmosis can be thought of as a diffusion of water down its concentration gradient. For example, if two compartments are separated by a membrane that is permeable to water but not to solute (say, our old friends ions $X^+$ and $Y^-$) and if the $X^+Y^-$ solution is placed on one side and water alone is placed on the other, something does happen. Water moves into the $X^+Y^-$ side.

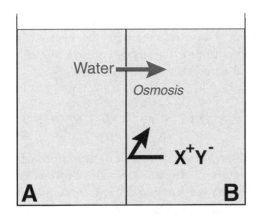

How much water will move? The net flow stops when the pressure created by the increase in fluid level on Side B (the hydrostatic pressure) equals the pressure drawing water out of Side A by osmosis (osmotic pressure).

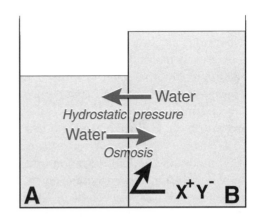

Let us return to capillary filtration. Only a small fraction of water moving out of the capillaries into the interstitial fluid is filtered. Most of it diffuses. What is filtered is pushed out by pressure in the capillary, which varies but is on average 32 mm Hg at the arteriole (front) end. This falls to about 15 mm Hg on the venule (back) end. Meanwhile, proteins in the blood, chiefly albumin, are essentially not filtered nor can they diffuse out of the capillary. These protein molecules exert an osmotic pressure that is about 25 mm Hg. This force tends to draw water into the vessel. (This may be called oncotic pressure or colloid osmotic pressure because it is the result of proteins suspended in blood.)

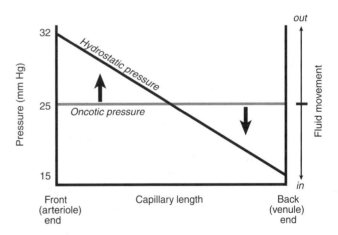

This means that at the front end of the capillary, hydrostatic pressure is greater than the osmotic pressure (by about 7 mm Hg). As a result, water with its small molecular constituents moves *out*. At the back end osmotic pressure is greater than hydrostatic pressure (by about 10 mm Hg) and water is drawn *back* into the capillary.

Albumin turns out to exert even more osmotic influence than one can account for solely on the basis of the number of its molecules held in a unit volume of plasma. Albumin binds a small number of $Cl^-$ ions, which in turn keep more $Na^+$ ions in the capillaries. This increase in electrolyte concentration increases the osmotic force attributable directly and indirectly to albumin.

This model of capillary filtration and adsorption is useful but not altogether accurate, given the complex arrangement of the capillary network. Actually, although filtration at one end of the capillary and absorption at the other do occur, more often some capillaries only filter and others only absorb. Also, some albumin does get out of the capillaries and not quite all of the filtered fluid gets reabsorbed. Both are picked up in the lymphatic vessels and ultimately return to the blood vessel system. (The lymphatic system, you recall, is the widely distributed network of small vessels that picks up the tissue fluid, with its constituents, that has not been returned by the capillaries to the circulatory system.)

Pinocytosis doesn't move many goods compared to diffusion or even to filtration, but it is an important and interesting process. Tiny vesicles filled with the molecules to be transported (often large and hydrophilic) are pinched off the endothelial cell membrane, move across the cell, and deliver their contents to the other side.

## ESPECIAL CELLS

So far we have seen capillaries accomplish very commendable work in the pickup and delivery of goods, all largely because of their simple structure and complex arrangement. What then makes the endothelial cell itself so praiseworthy? So what if it passively participates in diffusion and filtration, and adds a little pinocytosis? Where and what are those talents earlier alluded to?

The endothelial cell is in fact far from passive. It actively leads a variety of special, essential processes. Before spotlighting some of them, I want to make a point about organization, both of the endothelium and of this chapter.

Endothelial cells line the entire circulatory system. Even the heart's endocardial lining is part of this continuous layer. Why then is the discussion of this population of cells, widespread as they are, found in the chapter about capillaries? I can think of three reasons.

First, the capillaries harbor most of the endothelial cells because the capillary surface area is so large. Second, most of the special endothelial functions are concentrated in (but, granted, not confined to) capillaries and the adjacent arterioles and venules -- in what is often called the microcirculation. Third, though it's an imperfect fit, it is simply the best location for the topic. Endothelial cells don't neatly conform to our organizational construct of the circulatory system, serving as a good reminder that Nature really has no interest in or use for the schemes that we make up to try to understand her.

## SPECIALITY #1: VASOACTIVITIES

The endothelial cell is a source of substances that cause vascular smooth muscle contraction or relaxation. One of these, prostacyclin, is released in response to shear stress and causes smooth muscle relaxation. It also inhibits platelet plugging of small vessels. Prostacyclin, then, is an important member of the team responsible for keeping blood vessels open. (This important team, as we will see, is largely fielded by endothelial cells.)

Endothelial cells also make both the potent vasodilator, nitric oxide, and the potent vasoconstrictor, endothelin. The chief target for the vasoactivity of all these compounds is the smooth muscle cells of the arterioles and venules.

## SPECIALITY #2: ANGIOGENESIS

Blood vessels are able to sprout new branches under a number of conditions. This process, known as angiogenesis, is in large part led by endothelial cells. One probable stimulus for angiogenesis is persisting low tissue oxygen level. This induces cells in the area to release growth factors with acronyms like VEGF (vascular endothelial growth factor) and FGF (fibroblast growth factor). These induce protein-degrading enzymes to clear away cell basement membrane. Now endothelial cells can migrate from preexisting vessels into the tissue where they proliferate. They line up properly in response to adhesion promoting molecules on their cell surfaces. These *integrins*, as they are called, are also induced by the growth factors. As these new endothelial cells line up, they form tubules in response to another integrin. Next the fragile vessels are stabilized by special cells, pericytes, that the endothelial cells recruit.

A period of remodeling then takes place. Some vessels not protected by pericytes regress while others with protection mature. The new small vascular tree is pruned.

Just as there are promoters of new vessel formation, there have to be inhibitors to ensure that the process is not overdone. Some inhibitors act on the basement-membrane–degrading enzymes, others interfere with VEGF and FGF, and still others block integrins. There is also a specific protein called endostatin that blocks endothelial cell proliferation, and another called angiostatin that reduces the adenosine triphosphate (ATP) supply of endothelial cells. The whole act of angiogenesis is balanced and orderly, thanks to initiatives and responses of endothelial cells.

## SPECIALITY #3: WHITE BLOOD CELL TRAFFICKING

One of the best stories about endothelial cells has to do with their key role in control of white blood cell traffic. (For a very enlightening and clever discussion of this and of the whole immune system, see the first book in this series: *How the Immune System Works* by Lauren Sompayrac.)

Just for fun (and because it isn't a bad analogy) consider white blood cells as crime fighters. The crimes they deal with range from vandalism (damage to an area by trauma, for example) to invasion (infection in a tissue) to subversion (cancer). These policemen have various jobs, and some have previous job experience. Neutrophils are especially good at combating invasion by bacteria like *Staphylococcus.* Eosinophils and mast cells like to take on parasite invaders. Lymphocytes come in a variety of types. T-lymphocytes, for example, circulate from the bloodstream through tissues and back into the bloodstream, looking for foreign and domestic enemies, then mount an attack when they are found.

Endothelial cells are central players in this activity. They not only flag down white cells when they are needed but they help them stop and pass through the vessel wall on their way to the tissue in need.

Let us look first at how the endothelium calls one of the most active cops, the neutrophil. If inflammation occurs in tissue nearby, a variety of messenger proteins called *cytokines* are produced. These diffuse to a nearby vessel and induce the endothelial cell to make on its surface one of a family of adhesion molecules called *selectins*. The selectin molecules recognize sticky mucin-like molecules on the neutrophil. This interaction causes tethering of the cell to the wall of the vessel as the cell flows by. This binding occurs rapidly and briefly, causing the neutrophil to begin to slow down and roll along the vessel in the direction of flow.

At this point another kind of molecule triggers step two. One of a variety of molecules called *chemoattractants* or *chemokines* (these are also produced in the inflamed area), which has diffused to the endothelium, acts on the neutrophil and, taking advantage of a G-protein signaling pathway, induces the neutrophil to activate another kind of adhesion molecule on its surface, an *integrin*. This integrin binds to a special molecule on the endothelial surface called an intercellular adhesion molecule (ICAM) which has already been induced by one or more of the cytokines. This integrin–ICAM binding sticks the neutrophil to the endothelial surface. Responding further to the chemoattractant, the neutrophil migrates through the endothelial layer into the tissue area where it is needed. (A neutrophil is so sensitive to its chemoattractants that it can detect a concentration difference of 1% across its diameter and move steadily in the direction of the greater concentration.)

There are then three steps in this process, and the steps are sequential but overlapping. First, selectin and mucin-like molecules interact to set up white cell rolling. Second, a chemoattractant activates white cell integrin adhesiveness. Third, integrin–ICAM stops the rolling and allows the white cell to enter the tissue and to follow the chemoattraction.

Each of these steps has variations, so by varying which selectin, which chemoattractant, or which ICAM is expressed, different subsets (neutrophils, other granulocytes, monocytes, or lymphocytes)

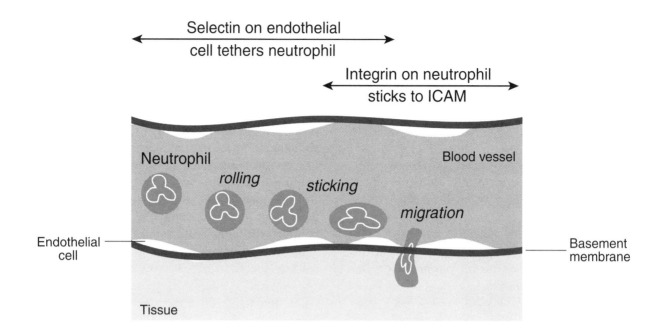

might be brought into the inflamed, infected, or invaded tissue. The endothelium can call the best cop for the job.

Calling in lymphocytes from the bloodstream to do surveillance or battle in the tissues is a very similar three-step process. Only here the endothelial cells can flag down specific lymphocyte groups to recirculate in the kinds of tissues where they had previously been activated and where they are most likely to find again their target enemy. The endothelial cells then recruit lymphocytes with previous experience dealing with crime in their particular neighborhood.

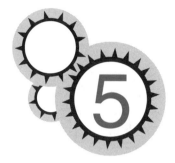

# THE VEINS

## REVIEW

Summary, please.

Capillaries, with their endothelial cells, deliver and pick up the goods by an assortment of schemes. Those goods may be smaller, like molecules of oxygen, or larger like neutrophils. Here smaller and larger, as comparative adjectives, are dramatically meaningful. There is a difference of four orders of magnitude, four powers of 10, between the diameters of an oxygen mole-cule and a neutrophil. It is as though your UPS carrier could deliver to you one of a pair of dice or the whole Las Vegas casino.

The remarkable versatility of capillaries and their endothelial cells makes them a key part in keeping all the body's cells tidy, happy, working, communicating, and safe.

What is Lecture 5 about? It is about the veins: they may be compliant, but they are not complaisant.

Whenever the parts of the circulatory system are described, veins always come last. They are what is left over; they complete the circuit, returning blood to the heart. But the venous system deserves better, as it has some very influential attributes.

## CAPACITY

Veins are capacitance vessels. They serve as a blood reservoir. At rest 60% of the body's total blood volume is in the veins. They can play this role because they are relatively thin-walled and, having little elastin and a thin muscular media, they are stretchable (that is, they have relatively high *compliance*) with little elastic recoil. Therefore, veins can accommodate a varying pool of blood.

Veins create little resistance because they have relatively large diameters. This is good because the pressure in the small veins (just where blood enters the venous system) is only 15 mm Hg. Right atrial pressure is about 0 mm Hg so there is a pressure difference of 15 mm Hg to drive the blood from the venules back to the heart. The volume of blood returned to the right atrium is called *venous return*.

Venous return can be enhanced. Sympathetic nervous system activity can cause veins to constrict, reducing the compliance of the system, and reducing the size of the reservoir. This also modestly raises the pressure in the venous system. With the increase in the pressure difference between the veins and the right atrium, venous return increases.

## THE VALUE OF VENOUS VALVES

Skeletal muscle activity also promotes venous return. As muscles in the arms and legs are active, they squeeze the veins so that intermittent contraction and relaxation of those muscles exerts a pumping action. This action squeezes the blood in only one direction, toward the heart, because valves placed intermittently inside the veins allow only one-way flow.

This mechanism is especially important in returning blood from the legs, as gravity tends to promote the pooling of blood in distensible leg veins. When a

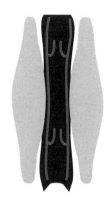

Muscle relaxed

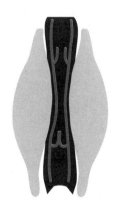

Muscle contracted

member of the Queen's Guard passes out after standing at rigid attention for a prolonged time, it is because he was not able to maintain enough venous return by contracting and relaxing his leg muscles.

Breathing also enhances blood return to the heart. On inspiration the chest cavity enlarges and the pressure inside falls below atmospheric pressure. That, of course, is why air enters the lungs. This same pressure drop also draws venous blood into the chest toward the heart.

And lastly, the heart itself adds to right atrial filling. With systole, the tricuspid valve is drawn down, "sucking" blood into the right atrium.

You may see a picture of venous pressure changes or pressure waves in large veins such as the jugular vein in the neck. When the right atrium contracts and when the tricuspid valve moves, a low magnitude wave -- rather like a ripple -- is sent out through the venous system. A pressure-detecting device in a vein can record such waves, and in fact they can sometimes be directly observed.

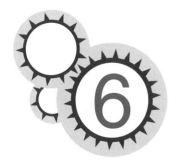

# THE BLOOD

Short lecture. Short summary?

Veins return blood to the heart. Like the other parts of the circulatory system, their design well serves their function. Veins are the circulatory system's capacitance vessels, and their capacity can be varied to adjust the rate of venous return. Flow of venous blood can also be enhanced by pumping action of surrounding skeletal muscles, by inspiration, and by cardiac systole.

What now? Now we come to the discussion of blood, the last of our circulatory system components. Blood is really a tissue -- a heterogenous, fluid tissue.

Blood is a complex tissue. It has both physiologic (or biologic) properties and physical (or mechanical) properties, which make it especially suited to be the transport medium of the circulatory system. The study of blood is a specialty unto itself, but we will select out some of its attributes that particularly tie it to the circulatory system's character and functions.

Blood consists of cells (red and white) and bits of cells (platelets) suspended in plasma. Plasma is a solution of salts, proteins, fats, carbohydrates, and gases. An average-sized person has 5 liters of blood -- about 55% of that is plasma and the rest is cells. There are about $5 \times 10^9$ red cells in each milliliter of blood.

## BLOOD BIOLOGIC

The physiologic topics included here are red cells' oxygen carrying and delivery, carbon dioxide exchange, and hemostasis (which includes blood clotting). We have already looked at white blood cell interactions with endothelial cells and plasma protein's role in capillary function.

## TAKING OXYGEN

Red blood cells are red because they have iron-containing molecules called heme, which can combine with oxygen ($O_2$). The heme molecules are attached to globin, a protein. Together they form hemoglobin which, strictly speaking, is the form without oxygen. Oxyhemoglobin is the proper name for the oxygenated form.

A major role of the circulatory system is to deliver oxygen to the body's cells, or more specifically to the mitochondria of the cells. It does this by passing the blood through the lungs where oxygen, abundant in the air in the lungs, diffuses into the blood and attaches to heme, with four oxygen molecules able to bind to each heme molecule.

One measure of the blood's oxygen level is the amount of oxygen combined with hemoglobin to form oxyhemoglobin. This is measured as the ratio of oxygen bound to hemoglobin to the total amount that can be bound. This is the *oxygen saturation* and is expressed as a percentage.

Another measure of oxygen in blood is its *partial pressure.* A mixture of gases, like air, exerts a pressure, whether it is confined in a tank made of steel or in the atmosphere by gravity. Each individual gas exerts part of that pressure -- that is, it exerts a partial pressure. At sea level, the partial pressure of oxygen, designated $PO_2$, is normally 21% of 760 mm Hg, or 160 mm Hg. When gases can dissolve in a liquid, they each exert individually a partial pressure there too. So oxygen has a partial pressure when it is dissolved in blood. Furthermore, a difference or gradient in the partial pressures of a gas causes it to diffuse from higher to lower partial pressure, or down the gradient. (Of course, if there is no gradient there is no net movement.)

There are important differences between oxygen saturation of hemoglobin and oxygen partial pressure in blood. Each represents a different form of oxygen in the blood. The first (oxygen saturation) is $O_2$ bound to hemoglobin and the second (partial pressure) is $O_2$ physically dissolved in plasma. The oxygen bound as oxyhemoglobin is not part of the partial pressure of oxygen. Still, these two are related.

That relationship between $PO_2$ and oxygen saturation is not linear. If you graph $PO_2$ against oxygen saturation you do not get a straight line. Instead you get an S-shaped curve, like this:

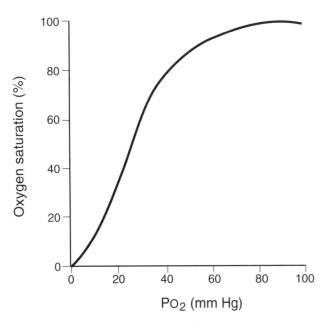

This shape results from the binding affinity heme has for all four of its oxygen molecules, which increases just as soon as the fourth one is in place. So it is harder to pull the first $O_2$ off. However, when it is off, the others follow more easily. This has fascinating consequences.

To appreciate those consequences let's look at the partial pressure gradients of oxygen going from ox-

ygen's source in the tiny air sacs of the lungs (each called an *alveolus*, a "small hollow") to its destination, the mitochondria of tissue cells. The $PO_2$ in the air in the alveoli is about 102 mm Hg. (All these numbers reflect sea level conditions.) Oxygen has only a very short diffusion distance to the blood and essentially loads up the hemoglobin. With a $PO_2$ of 95 mm Hg of the blood in the capillaries leaving the alveoli, the hemoglobin is nearly 100% saturated, so even with a higher $PO_2$ very little more oxygen would be accommodated, especially as oxygen doesn't dissolve very well in plasma. There is little change in blood $PO_2$ during its travel in the arteries. Even if there were to be a drop to 70 mm Hg, little oxygen would have been given up by hemoglobin because this range of 70 to 95 mm Hg is on the "flat" part of the curve. Once in the capillary, the fall in blood $PO_2$ is well into the "steep" part, with hemoglobin dumping off oxygen with any reduction in $PO_2$. This, of course, is fitting. You don't want to spill your cargo en route; instead you want to arrive at your destination with as full a load as possible. Oxygen, duly delivered, diffuses down its partial pressure gradient from about 55 mm Hg (which is average in a capillary though this falls to 40 mm Hg at its end) to the cell with its mitochondria where, at rest, the $PO_2$ is about 10 mm Hg.

Note that as the blood leaves the systemic capillary it still has a $PO_2$ of 40 mm Hg, which means that it is still 75% saturated with oxygen. What kind of system is this that makes its delivery and then leaves still carrying 75% of its goods? It is an especially well-designed system because the surplus guards against running low when the cells' demand for oxygen increases. It is better to hold on to some oxygen, even a lot, and continue to circulate with it than to be caught short. The tissue cells at some point will be called into action and start to use more oxygen. As their $PO_2$ falls to 5 or even to 1 mm Hg, mitochondria can carry out oxidative metabolism.

One aside is illustrative. If blood did not have hemoglobin, it could hold about 3 mL of oxygen in each liter at a $PO_2$ of 100 mm Hg. (One mL of oxygen is the amount of oxygen -- the number of $O_2$ molecules -- that would occupy 1 mL at sea level.) With cardiac output of 5 L/min, the circulatory system could supply the body with only 15 mL of oxygen each minute. At resting conditions the body's cells need 250 mL of $O_2$ each minute and this need can go up as high as 12 times that during strenuous exercise. At that high level of need, without hemoglobin in the blood, the heart would have to pump 1000 liters of blood a minute. You and I would be, I think, all heart.

## RETURNING CARBON DIOXIDE

The transport of carbon dioxide ($CO_2$) from tissue capillaries to lung capillaries also has some special features. Carbon dioxide is 20 times more soluble in plasma than is oxygen, so while some $CO_2$ does dissolve in blood, it is still a small part of the total transported. Another relatively small part binds reversibly with hemoglobin and plasma proteins making so-called carbamino compounds. Most $CO_2$ is converted inside red cells into carbonic acid by the enzyme carbonic anhydrase (CA).

$$CO_2 + H_2O \leftrightarrow H_2CO_3$$

This rapidly dissociates into $H^+$ and $HCO_3^-$. The bicarbonate ion ($HCO_3^-$) diffuses out of the red cell in exchange for $Cl^-$ which comes in from the plasma. Most of the $H^+$ produced quickly combines, again reversibly, with hemoglobin.

This all occurs in the tissue capillaries where $CO_2$ has followed its partial pressure gradient. (The $P_{CO_2}$ in tissues is about 50; in capillary blood it's about 44.) These reactions all reverse in the pulmonary capillaries where blood $P_{CO_2}$ falls to about 40 mm Hg as $CO_2$ is given up to the air in the lungs.

Notice again that not nearly all of the systemic venous $CO_2$ is off-loaded to the alveolar air. The body requires a large amount of $CO_2$ in the blood to maintain its normal concentration of $H^+$ -- that is, its normal pH.

Hemoglobin has another elegant trick. Its affinity for oxygen goes down when it is exposed to relatively acidic conditions. As a result, while $CO_2$ and its product carbonic acid are rising in the systemic capillaries, oxygen release is enhanced by as much as 10%. The converse of this process takes place in the pulmonary capillaries, increasing oxygen uptake by hemoglobin.

## STASIS

Hemostasis literally means "blood standing still" and it is a wonderful word for our next topic in blood physiology. The circulatory system can reduce and even stop blood's escaping from holes in blood ves-

sels, and it can also plug those holes. It can indeed make blood stand still. Hemostasis is really three processes: vasoconstriction, platelet plugging, and blood coagulation or clotting.

If a blood vessel is opened up, the smooth muscle in its wall will contract, narrowing or even closing the vessel. The contraction results from a number of influences -- direct mechanical stimulation, local sympathetic nerve stimulation, and the action of compounds like endothelin and serotonin released in the area. (Serotonin, derived from the amino acid tryptophan, is often called into service by the body. It not only has vasoactive duties when released from platelets, but also acts in the central and peripheral nervous systems as a neurotransmitter.)

Platelet plugging of a tear in a small blood vessel is the first step in blood clotting. Platelets are cell fragments, pieces of a bone marrow cell called the megakaryocyte which sheds these bits of its cytoplasm into the bloodstream. (Megakaryocytes are indeed large cells just as their name says. When stimulated they replicate their chromosomes without dividing, a process that can yield a cell with a chromosome count as high as $32n$.)

Small as platelets are -- less than half the diameter of a red cell -- they are a biochemical treasure chest. On a platelet's surface is an array of those adhesive molecules, integrins. Integrins are glycoproteins (part protein, part sugar) and, you recall, they determine how cells, or in this case pieces of cells, stick together or stick to extracellular structural molecules. The integrin of most interest here is called glycoprotein (GP) IIb/IIIa (this is just a way to code these molecules by their structures). There are probably 60,000 copies of it on each platelet and when the platelet is "resting" (circulating freely) GP IIb/IIIa is also inactive. When vascular injury occurs and the endothelium is broken through, platelets are exposed to, and may bind to, a number of substances that are in the underlying tissue or are released into the area. Those substances include ADP, epinephrine, collagen, and thrombin (more on this enzyme later). Any of them can signal a change (G proteins again) that activates platelets. The GP IIb/IIIa's become sticky. They bind a protein, fibrinogen, that forms a bridge between platelets linking IIb/IIIa on one platelet to IIb/IIIa on another. This linking causes aggregation of a large number of platelets at the site of injury.

Activated platelets secrete several substances. One, thromboxane $A_2$, produces vasoconstriction and also promotes platelet clumping. Others are serotonin, of course; adhesive proteins to reinforce the platelet plug; and even growth factors to begin mediating tissue repair.

Released from the site of tissue trauma or exposure is a glycoprotein called "tissue factor," which starts a series of reactions, each of which is a conversion of a proenzyme to an active enzyme which then catalyzes the next step. This process is promoted by the activated platelets that assemble the participating compounds. The result is the formation of the enzyme thrombin (from its precursor, prothrombin). In this scheme thrombin does two things from here. It starts a side chain of reactions that doubles back to amplify its own formation. It also performs the last act of the series -- cleaving fibrinogen so that its pieces can reassemble to make fibrin. Fibrin molecules, strung together and cross-linked, form the jelly-like clot that overlies the damaged area.

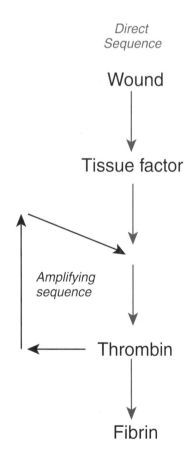

*Direct Sequence*

## Wound

## Tissue factor

*Amplifying sequence*

## Thrombin

## Fibrin

It should come as no surprise that for each step in this scheme there is a counter move that the body uses to modify, reduce, or stop these processes. A blood clot in the right place and of the right size is one thing;

recurring clotting or a clot in the wrong place is dangerous.

Endothelin and thromboxane $A_2$ are opposed in arteries by nitric oxide (NO) released by the endothelium. The NO causes vasodilatation and reduces platelet aggregation. Prostacyclin, another vasodilator that comes from endothelial cells (as we have already seen), also counters platelet aggregation. It is interesting to note that prostacyclin and thromboxane $A_2$, which have directly opposing actions, are both synthesized from the same fatty acid-derived molecule, arachidonic acid.

Thrombin and another key enzyme in the clotting scheme are inhibited -- immediately and irreversibly -- by a circulating peptide, antithrombin III (AT-III), when it is teamed up with heparin, a polysaccharide present in many tissues. I mention this for two reasons. First, heparin is commonly used as a drug to prevent clotting. Second, endothelial cell surfaces are normally coated with a layer of AT-III, bound and activated by a cell surface heparin-like substance, and ready to take out any thrombin that happens to float by.

Another clot-inhibiting operative acts on thrombin. The protein thrombomodulin is found in the cell membrane of endothelial cells of small vessels. It is located on the lumen side and it, of course, reacts with thrombin. It does not inactivate thrombin, but rather alters it so that thrombin no longer makes fibrin or activates platelets. In this new form, sitting on the endothelial cell, thrombin now activates an enzyme that destroys two of the clotting factors. Thrombin has been turned and is now in the anticoagulant camp.

Finally, there is another inhibitor that acts very early in the clotting scheme. This tissue factor pathway inhibitor (TFPI) is also made by endothelial cells of small vessels and sits on their surfaces. It is active after heparin releases it into the blood.

It occurs to me that I might have changed the emphasis of this subsection and put it among the list of endothelial cell specialties with the label "Avoiding Stasis." For we see how active endothelial cells, especially those of small blood vessels, are in trying to keep blood vessels open and clot free. Endothelial cells strive not to make blood stand still, but to make blood flow.

Fortunately, clots do form when necessary. Following the formation of a proper clot it undergoes molding. It shrinks or retracts, drawing the borders of the injured area closer together. This is accomplished by platelets caught up in the clot. Their activated GP IIb/

IIIa integrin causes the clumping, and signals the platelet to contract. And what is there in a platelet to contract? Yes, actin and myosin.

The clot or thrombus plays a key role but there comes a time when it is no longer needed. Blood flow needs to be restored. The body anticipates this by initiating the process of clot removal virtually as soon as it is formed. The clot is lysed or broken down by another series of enzymatic reactions. The fibrinolytic (fibrin dissolving) process begins with conversion of plasminogen to plasmin. This conversion is catalyzed in blood vessels by tissue plasminogen activator (tPA) and in tissues outside blood vessels by urokinase. Plasmin then "digests" or breaks down the mesh of fibrin, cutting it into small pieces.

## BLOOD MECHANICAL

The physical or mechanical properties of blood affect how it flows. Blood is a complex fluid. Because it is a suspension of the formed elements, cells and platelets, it is not homogeneous. Blood is also a variable fluid. For example, the total and relative amounts of many of the plasma proteins can change. Although this complexity and variability reflect the many functions blood performs so well, they also influence how it flows.

As an illustration of a complicated property of blood, let us use its viscosity. Newton defined it very specifically, but for our purposes viscosity is qualitatively defined as a fluid's "internal friction." It is one of the factors that determine resistance to the flow of any fluid. Viscosity also helps determine *how* a fluid flows.

It is to the body's advantage for blood to flow, as much as possible, in a streamlined fashion. This so-called *laminar flow* can be visualized as being made up of tiny cylindrical layers of fluid beginning with the layer right next to the vessel wall. Flow there is apt to be slow because of the drag created by the wall; that layer may be nearly motionless. The next fluid layer moves a little faster, and so on, with the middle part moving fastest. Each layer slips by its exterior layer smoothly with less and less drag as the layers approach the middle. Laminar flow is the most efficient arrangement of fluid movement. Contrast this with turbulent flow where there is no streamlining but instead multiple vortices of tumbling fluid in the vessel. This chaotic pattern requires a much greater pressure to achieve a given flow than does the laminar arrangement.

It turns out that laminar flow can best be maintained by not letting the fluid viscosity get too low. It is also apt to be maintained by slow flow rate, low fluid density, and small tube diameter. In addition it helps to avoid abrupt changes in vessel diameter and to keep the vessel walls smooth.

Viscosity then can't be too high since that would create excessive resistance, or too low because that would contribute to causing turbulent flow. There is still another twist.

Viscosity of blood is not fixed. It is different in different parts of the circulatory system and can change as blood constituents change. For one thing, viscosity of blood varies depending on how many red cells are in it. Red cell count in blood is often expressed as *hematocrit*, which is the ratio of red cell volume to the volume of whole blood. The usual hematocrit is 40% to 50%. As the hematocrit increases, blood viscosity increases, raising resistance. Consequently, the work of the heart needed to pump the blood increases. But as the hematocrit decreases, the number of red cells is less and consequently the work of the heart increases as it has to pump more volume of blood to carry adequate oxygen to the body's cells. So there is an ideal hematocrit level that can be calculated, which balances these conflicting variables. What is it? 40 to 50!

Viscosity can also change with vessel diameter. In small vessels the red cells tend to flow in the middle and flow faster than outer plasma layers. This increases the relative amount of the slower going plasma, and thus in effect *lowers* the hematocrit in the vessel. This helps to offset the next (and the last) variable.

Viscosity of blood is greater when flow rate is less. In part this is because red cells tend to clump together at low flow rates. This clumping can be aggravated by high concentration of certain proteins in the blood, especially fibrinogen.

So how do red cells, at times even clumped, get through these small capillaries? Red cells are biconcave discs -- with greater surface area to volume ratio than spheres -- that are *flexible*. They are easily bent and folded, and able to slide through an opening as small as 3 μm when their diameter in their usual shape is 7 μm.

# SPECIAL CIRCULATIONS

## 7

## REVIEW

So what are the key points?

Blood is best viewed not just as a passive liquid into which are dissolved molecules that the cells of the body need or want to get rid of. Although this is blood's role in part, more accurately blood is an active tissue that fulfills its multiple roles by being (usually) fluid in form --

an admirable complicated form -- and by having special schemes for carrying and delivering things like oxygen, carbon dioxide, and white blood cells. It is a coequal partner with all the other parts of the circulatory system.

We know all the players now. How about some stories? Here are some vascular tales with a moral: all circulations are special.

How nature deals with special situations and solves problems is always fascinating, and never more so than when we consider some of the special arrangements for circulation that the human body has contrived. With unique variations of common components, nature can mold parts of the circulatory system to fit any organ's or tissue's needs perfectly.

We begin with an example of molding the system to meet an entire individual's needs. That individual is an unborn baby and that molding is the fetal circulation.

## FETAL CIRCULATION -- VERY SPECIAL

You know the situation: in the uterus the infant receives its oxygen and nutrients from the mother through the placenta. There is no air in the baby's lungs and the baby's heart is actively circulating the blood. All the nutrient rich, oxygenated blood comes from the placenta via the umbilical vein and passes into the baby's systemic venous circulation. Those parts of the developing body with the greatest need for this blood -- with the greatest metabolic activity -- are the brain, the heart, and the liver. So the question is, what kind of scheme can

deliver the goods to the whole body, but preferentially to where those goods are needed the most?

The umbilical vein carries blood to the liver where half of it flows through the liver via the portal vein and the other half bypasses the liver by going through the ductus venosus into the infant's inferior vena cava, mixing with blood from the lower trunk and legs. A short distance later it is joined with blood from the liver coming into the inferior vena cava from the hepatic veins. There is very incomplete mixing in the inferior vena cava, with the two streams running side by side. The larger parallel stream, which is chiefly umbilical vein blood, goes to the right atrium and tends to be shunted through the atrial septum to the left atrium through a hole, the foramen ovale. This is really a kind of flap valve held open by the constant flow of blood from the right atrium to the left atrium.

The other parallel stream reaches the right atrium and, mixing with blood from the upper body (delivered to the right atrium by the superior vena cava), goes to the right ventricle. It is then pumped out into the pulmonary artery. In the fetus, pulmonary vascular resistance is quite high (the arterioles have a thick media), so 90% of the right ventricular blood goes not to the lungs, but rather through the ductus arteriosus, which is a shunt from the pulmonary artery to the aorta.

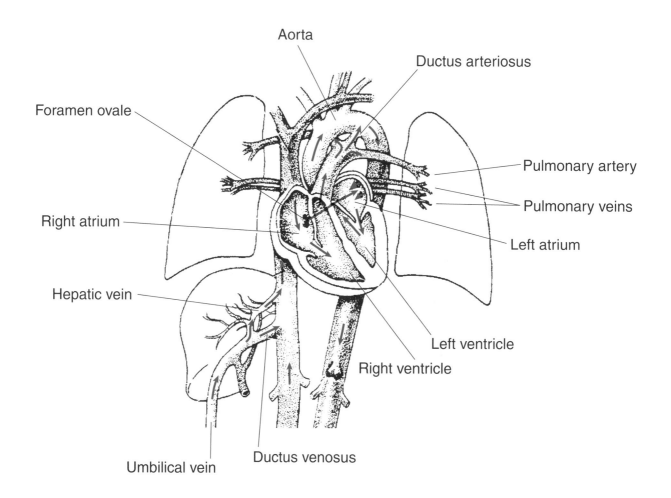

The ductus arteriosus joins the aorta beyond the origin of the arteries that supply the head and arms.

The large amount of blood passing through the foramen ovale joins the small amount returning from the lungs. This left atrial blood then fills the left ventricle and is pumped into the aorta. Most of that blood goes to the head, arms, and upper thorax. The rest joins the blood coming through the ductus arteriosus and supplies the rest of the body, including the umbilical arteries which return blood to the placenta.

If you haven't already, take a minute to trace these pathways in the picture. Note that in this arrangement the heart's two pumps act not in series, but in parallel. In fact, the right ventricle pumps more blood, up to two times more, than the left ventricle pumps.

The placental membranes do not allow equilibration of the partial pressure of oxygen ($P_{O_2}$) between the maternal and fetal circulations. As a consequence the $P_{O_2}$ of the oxygenated fetal blood is low. But the special hemoglobin of the fetus has such a high affinity for oxygen that it can carry it in high amount even at relatively low $P_{O_2}$.

With this arrangement of fetal circulation, oxygen and nutrients are delivered as needed for the baby's healthy prenatal development. Birth sets off a series of interlocking events. The umbilical vessels are either tied off or spasm shut, raising the baby's peripheral resistance and systemic blood pressure. The ductus venosus automatically closes because no blood is flowing from the umbilical vein. The lungs fill with air and pulmonary vascular resistance falls by about 90%. (More gradually, over a few weeks the pulmonary arterioles undergo thinning of their muscular media.)

With the increase in blood flow through the lungs and into the left atrium and the reduction of flow into the right atrium (again because of occlusion of the umbilical vein), the foramen ovale closes and soon fuses over. One or two days after birth, the ductus arteriosus closes completely. The heart is now two pumps aligned in series. The lifelong configuration of the circulatory system is established.

Before discussing examples of special tissue and organ circulation, I will remind you that each special area enjoys a considerable amount of autonomy in regulating its own blood flow. That autonomy may be overridden to ensure the body's greater good, but the arrangement of having circulations connected in parallel usually gives each special circulation essentially the same blood pressure difference (between mean arterial pressure and venous pressure) to use to create flow. How much flow will depend on the amount of resistance the special area chooses to have.

## THE BRAIN -- TOP PRIORITY

Consider the brain. It needs a constant, unfailing blood supply. Even 5 seconds of interruption in circulation to the brain causes loss of consciousness, and a few minutes results in permanent tissue damage. Because the brain is enclosed in a rigid confined space, the volume of blood going in must equal that coming out. Any increase in volume of fluid in the cranium, as occurs with brain swelling, raises the pressure in this closed space and may hinder incoming blood flow.

The rate of cerebral blood flow is remarkably constant -- around 55 mL/minute/100 gram brain tissue. Even if the mean arterial blood pressure varies between 60 and 160 mm Hg, this flow rate is kept steady, thanks (probably) to the myogenic mechanism of autoregulation. There is, however, an increase in blood flow to local areas in the brain where greater neuronal activity is taking place. This is all largely mediated by metabolic factors ($K^+$ and $H^+$) and adenosine.

Blood supply to the brain is made more secure by a special arterial arrangement. Four arteries in the neck -- two carotids in the front and two vertebrals in the back -- comprise the brain's source of blood. The vertebrals join to become the basilar artery which, at the base of the brain, forms an arterial ring with the two carotid arteries. From this ring, known as the circle of Willis, the specific cerebral arteries arise. If one (and sometimes even up to three) of the four arteries is occluded, flow from the remaining ones (or one) is available.

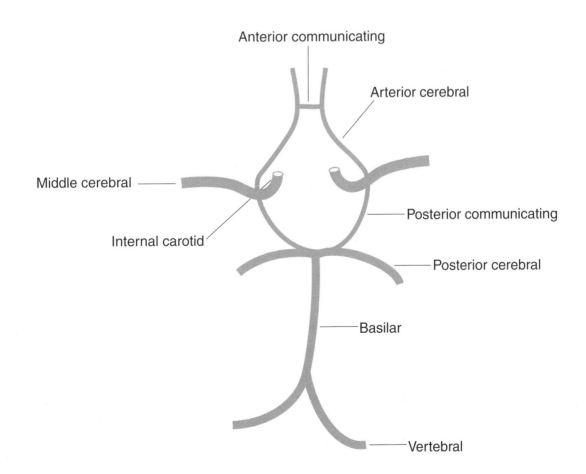

The blood–brain barrier helps protect brain tissue from metabolic imbalance and from toxins. This barrier is a complex of devices that limits what can pass from the blood to brain cells. The endothelial cells of brain capillaries have tight junctions without pores between them and a dense basement membrane beneath them. Also these cells are rich in mitochondria to support high metabolic activity and in enzymes to degrade unwanted molecules. Then there are special brain cells called glial cells that abut on the basement membrane so there is essentially no extracellular space in the brain into which unwanted molecules can diffuse.

## THE HEART -- SELF-SERVICE

It is fitting and proper that the heart, like the brain, receives preferential treatment. The heart is intolerant of any interruption of its blood supply (because it functions only aerobically). Its need for blood varies greatly because its workload changes so much.

Coronary blood flow is largely controlled by local factors (probably chiefly adenosine) and not by humeral or neural factors. As the heart's oxygen demand increases, so does coronary blood flow, up to five times its basal rate. It is true that with sympathetic stimulation there is an increase in coronary blood flow, but this occurs as an indirect result of faster heart rate and greater force of contraction, both of which cause an increase in oxygen demand.

The heart is in the unique situation of generating its own blood flow and it must do this while intermittently contracting and relaxing. During systole the contracting myocardium squeezes down on the vessels that course through it. In fact, during early systole the blood flow in arteries to the left ventricle stops or even reverses direction briefly. Maximal left coronary inflow has to occur during early diastole when there is no compression of the arteries.

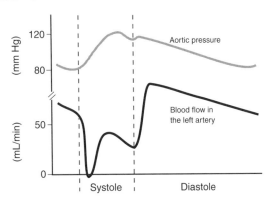

## SKIN -- INTERFACING

Skin has a relatively small need for nutrients and oxygen but its circulation serves the important function of helping maintain constant body temperature. When heat dissipation is needed, blood flow to the skin is increased; when heat conservation is needed, blood flow is decreased. The changes in flow can be amplified by specially designed arteriolar shunts between arterioles and venules, bypassing their capillary beds. When opened, these shunts bring more blood to the skin surface than would be made possible by dilatation of the standard precapillary arterioles.

The regulation of these skin vessels is chiefly neural. Reflex sympathetic activity is modulated by changes in ambient and internal body temperatures. The temperature sensing and regulating center in the brain is in the hypothalamus.

## LIVER -- TWICE TENDED

The liver gets most of its blood (75%) from the portal vein which receives blood from the alimentary tract. The blood brings the variety of goods, including nutrients absorbed from the gut, to the liver where these compounds are used, stored, circulated, or detoxified.

The liver obviously needs another blood supply, an arterial blood supply, to bring oxygen. This is provided by the hepatic artery. This combination of arterial and venous flow gives the liver about 25% of the cardiac output.

The two blood sources run side by side in the liver as they give rise to smaller and smaller branches. These two sets of branches run through the liver tissue. Blood from both ends up in the hepatic venules. The capillaries between the portal venules and the hepatic venules have discontinuous endothelial cells. This allows the liver cells access to essentially everything in the blood except blood cells. The hepatic venules come together to constitute the hepatic veins, which empty into the inferior vena cava.

Note that the liver has a so-called "portal circulation" with a capillary bed between two venous systems, the portal vein and the hepatic veins. Blood circulating to the intestinal tract then has two "capillary experiences," one in the intestinal tract and one in the liver. In the first capillary bed it picks up nutrients, and

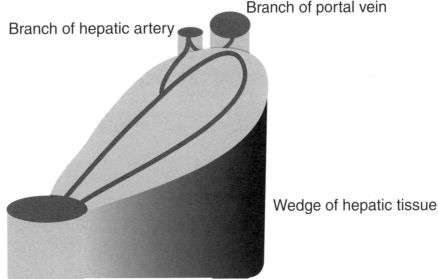

Branch of hepatic artery    Branch of portal vein

Wedge of hepatic tissue

Branch of hepatic vein

in the second it delivers them to or transports them from liver cells.

## KIDNEY -- FINE FILTERING

The kidney circulation provides the means of filtering the blood. Blood comes into each kidney via its renal artery. This breaks down into small arterioles called afferent ("carrying to") arterioles. Each afferent arteriole feeds a tuft of capillaries, which is surrounded by a tubule that collects what is filtered out. That filtrate is essentially plasma without proteins. The endothelium of these capillaries is fenestrated, which helps promote the escape of fluid and small molecules. These filtering units are called glomeruli ("little balls"). From each glomerulus another arteriole is reformed from the capillaries.

This second arteriole, the efferent ("carrying from"), leads to a second capillary bed, this one surrounding the tubule carrying the filtrate. By a number of wonderful tactics these capillaries (which also have fenestrated endothelium) recover those things -- like water, ions, and glucose -- that the body needs; and they recover them in the necessary amount. The rest is excreted as urine.

Note that here again we see two sets of capillary beds, but this time separated not by veins but by arterioles. Having arterioles (with all their flow-regulating capabilities) on both sides of the glomerulus allows the filtering pressure in the glomerular capillaries to be finely varied.

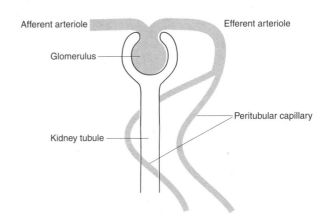

Afferent arteriole    Efferent arteriole

Glomerulus

Peritubular capillary

Kidney tubule

## LUNG -- PROPER PRESSURE

The pulmonary circulation takes unoxygenated blood in its arteries to small capillaries surrounding the alveoli. There the blood in those capillaries gives up carbon dioxide and takes on oxygen. The air in the alveoli is moved in and out by breathing, of course.

The lungs need another source of blood to bring oxygen and nutrients for their own metabolism. The systemic circulation provides bronchial arteries to do just that.

As we have noted the pulmonary circulation is a low pressure system (compared to the systemic circulation), with pulmonary artery pressure usually 24/9 mm Hg and mean arterial pressure 14 mm Hg. As a result, the osmotic pressure in the alveolar capillaries (still about 25 mm Hg) is much greater than the hydrostatic pressure (10.5 mm Hg). This keeps capillary fluid from leaking into the air sacs where it would interfere with gas exchange.

One might conclude that herein we have a reason for two circulations, one high pressure and one low pressure. For in the high pressure systemic circulation, capillary pressure needs to be high enough *to push fluid out* into the tissues; and in the low pressure pulmonary circulation, capillary pressure needs to be low enough that the prevailing osmotic pressure can *prevent fluid from being pushed out* into the alveoli.

Among the factors that control blood flow within the lung is oxygen level. In the *pulmonary* circulation an area of lower oxygenation causes vasoconstriction, shunting blood away. This keeps pulmonary arterial blood, which is already unoxygenated, from going through an area where it cannot receive oxygen. If this were to happen, the poorly oxygenated blood would end up in the general circulation, ''diluting down'' the arterial oxygen saturation.

On the other hand, a low oxygen level causes vasodilation in the *bronchial* arteries bringing more blood to an area that is likely to have low oxygen because of inflammation due to injury or infection.

# COUPLING HEART AND VESSELS

## 8

## REVIEW

What is the lesson from Lecture 7?

"Special circulation" is really a misleading term, because there is no true "general circulation." There are no general or generic cells in the body. Each cell is part of a tissue or organ with a specific set of functions, and with specific requirements from the circulatory system. It is wondrous that this one system, by modifying its basic parts, can serve so many disparate functions of cells -- be they processors, filterers, movers, storers, or cogitators.

Where to now? The next lecture is about appreciating the circulatory system as an entity, a functioning unit.

---

Having started with an overview of the circulatory system, we then looked at what we defined as its pieces and at variations and special arrangements of those pieces. Now we will look at the circulatory system assembled and how the heart and vessels are coupled, not anatomically, but functionally, to work as a unit. The first question will be, at the most fundamental level, *how* does this system *fit together*? The second question will be, *how* does this system *work*, in all its integrated complexity?

## WHENCE CARDIAC OUTPUT?

If the circulatory system is to get blood close to each cell in the body, it has to move enough blood to do it. The blood it moves is the cardiac output. There are four factors that determine cardiac output. They are heart rate, myocardial contractility, preload, and afterload. The first two originate *in* the heart alone (although they are affected by neural and humoral influences outside the heart).

Preload and afterload are the result of forces acting *on* the heart. Remember that preload is the volume of blood in the ventricle at the end of filling; it is the workload impressed on the heart just *before*

contraction begins. Afterload is the aortic pressure against which the heart must work to open the aortic valve; it is the workload impressed on the heart just *after* it starts to contract. Because afterload affects cardiac output essentially by influencing preload (if you want to review this, see Chapter 2), we will focus on the latter.

Preload is especially important because it is not only a *determinant of* cardiac output; it is also *determined by* cardiac output. To clarify this let's use a model of the circulatory system. This particular model has four parts. We lump the heart and pulmonary circulation together and call it a pump-oxygenator. Then there is the arterial system (arteries down to but not including arterioles). Third is the high-resistance microcirculation (arterioles, along with capillaries and venules) which creates peripheral resistance. And then comes the venous system (all the veins after the venules).

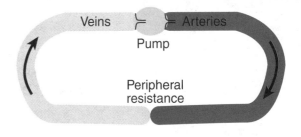

The arterial component is not very compliant. Although compliance is a description of how loose or pliable the walls of a vessel are, it also has a quantitative definition. It is the ratio of volume change to pressure change (dV/dP). The compliance of the veins is 19 times greater than that of the arteries. Arteries are stiff; veins are baggy.

So first we have the pump-oxygenator, then the stiff arteries. Third comes the resistance area through which the blood must be pushed, and then the compliant veins that hold most of the blood in the system.

## CENTRAL INDEED

Now let's add a key measurement, central venous pressure (CVP). This is the pressure at the end of the systemic venous line just where blood is returned to the heart (or pump oxygenator). This is also, in our model, preload because it determines ventricular filling. In the real biologic system (not the model) it is right atrial and right ventricular end-diastolic pressure.

Just as cardiac output can be affected by a number of factors, so can central venous pressure. Both an increase in blood volume and an increase in venous vasoconstriction (reducing the compliance of the veins) raise CVP. Also arteriolar dilatation will increase CVP because some additional amount of blood on the arterial side is allowed through to enter the veins. Of course, changes in the opposite directions -- reduced blood level, increased venous compliance, or increased arteriolar vasoconstriction -- all lower CVP.

What happens to cardiac output as you vary central venous pressure? Because central venous pressure represents ventricular filling and because of the Frank-Starling mechanism (you remember -- if you stretch cardiac muscle fibers they contract with more force), raising central venous pressure (stretching those myocardial fibers) raises cardiac output. Conversely, lowering central venous pressure lowers cardiac output. In this way central venous pressure and cardiac output are *directly* related.

$$\uparrow CVP \rightarrow \uparrow CO$$

What if, instead of first changing central venous pressure, you first change cardiac output? What if you raise cardiac output, for example? Then CVP goes *down*. And if you lower cardiac output, then CVP goes *up*.

Now we have cardiac output and central venous pressure being *inversely* related. This makes sense because by increasing CO you are taking more blood from the venous side and putting it into the arterial side. And it doesn't just transfer around to the venous side immediately because the resistance vessels of the microcirculation are in the way.

We can understand this better by looking at an extreme case. Let's say the system, as in the model, is humming along. We'll put in some typical numbers. The pump oxygenator (heart) is pumping 5 liter/minute. The pressure on the arterial side averages 102 mm Hg and the pressure on the venous side (the CVP) averages 2 mm Hg. The resistance is calculated then as:

$$\frac{102 - 2}{5}$$

(pressure difference over flow) or 20 mm Hg/liter/minute.

Now stop the pump. No more blood flows through the heart. (Assume the resistance stays the same.) As long as there is a pressure difference between the arterial side and venus side, blood will flow into the veins, and the venous side will continue to fill.

When, or where, will the pressure on the two sides be equal? The answer is *not* when the pressure on the two sides reaches an average (102 + 2)/2, or 52 mm Hg.

Because the veins are so compliant, so baggy (19 times more so than the arteries) the two pressures will equalize only when the arterial side pressure has fallen 19 times more than the venous side pressure has increased. So blood will flow through the resistance vessels until each side is at a pressure of 7 mm Hg. Why? Because CVP will have gone from 2 mm Hg to 7 mm Hg, a 5 mm Hg rise. The arterial side will have fallen from 102 mm Hg to 7 mm Hg, or 95 mm Hg. And 95 mm Hg is 19 times more than the 5 mm Hg change in CVP.

We can see that in this extreme situation a lot of blood has flowed into the venous side. And we can better understand why a fall in cardiac output (not as drastic as in the example) will raise the CVP, even if a relatively small amount. Conversely, a rise in cardiac output (CO) will lower the CVP.

$$\uparrow CO \rightarrow \downarrow CVP$$

## STABILITY, SOUGHT AND FOUND

Combining these two relationships we get:

$$\uparrow CVP \rightarrow \uparrow CO \rightarrow \downarrow CVP \rightarrow \downarrow CO$$

Cardiac output and CVP modulate each other. They keep each other in line and give the circulatory system stability.

Consider the other possibilities. What if raising the CO raised the CVP? (This could happen if there was no high-resistance microcirculation, for example.) Then,

$$\uparrow CVP \rightarrow \uparrow CO \rightarrow \uparrow CVP \rightarrow \uparrow CO$$

The upward spiral would accelerate the system out of control.

And what if raising CVP caused a reduction in CO? (This might happen if the heart running at capacity, without a Frank-Starling mechanism, had an increase in preload.) Then,

$$\uparrow CVP \rightarrow \downarrow CO \rightarrow \uparrow CVP \rightarrow \downarrow CO$$

Cardiac output would slow to a trickle.

The system that does exist might be considered to be at risk also. Great oscillations -- large swings in CVP and CO -- would negate much of its stabilizing influence. That risk is essentially removed by two factors. First, the increase in force of contraction induced by stretching ventricular myocardial fibers is limited and therefore the resulting increase in cardiac output is limited. Second, as we see in the model, the reduction in CVP from increasing CO is not great because of the low compliance of the veins.

The system is able to achieve stability. It is able to reach a point of equilibrium, which at rest is a cardiac output of about 5 liter/minute and a CVP of about 2 mm Hg. Even when the physiologic state of the system changes from a resting mode, the result is not chaos but merely a new equilibrium point.

Many of those other influences on CO and on CVP can alter that set point of equilibrium. Take, for example, myocardial contractility. If this is enhanced by sympathetic stimulation, the CO is increased. There is some net transfer of blood from the compliant venous side to the stiff arterial side of the circuit. The resulting fall in CVP will cause some reduction in CO but not enough to offset the induced increase. A new set point

will be established where CO is somewhat higher and CVP is a bit lower.

What if total peripheral resistance is raised? This raises afterload. As a result cardiac output goes down. This is temporarily compensated for by an increase in preload. However, over the long run this lowers CO (because the heart has an ongoing increased workload). Because increased total peripheral resistance causes more blood to be held in the arterial side of the circuit, CVP tends to be lowered unless the reduction in cardiac output is too great. It looks like this:

$$\uparrow TPR \rightarrow \downarrow CO \rightarrow \uparrow CVP$$
$$\searrow \downarrow CVP$$

So, increasing total peripheral resistance can result in higher or lower central venous pressure.

What if cardiac contractility is reduced? Tracing over our steps from the previous discussion about increased myocardial contractility, we can reason that here the set point would be one at which the CO is down and the CVP is up. Now let's add an increase in blood volume to the situation. (This is in fact what happens in heart failure. Myocardial contractility goes down and blood volume does increase because fluid is retained by the kidneys and by the action of elevated levels of the adrenal hormone aldosterone.) This increases CVP further but it also allows some restoration of CO, a tradeoff that is at least temporarily advantageous.

$$\downarrow CO \rightarrow \uparrow CVP \rightarrow \uparrow\uparrow CVP \rightarrow \uparrow CO$$
$$\nearrow$$
$$\uparrow blood\ volume$$

So however the equilibrium point may vary, it is still a set of conditions around which the heart and vessels can organize their performance. I think we have answered our first question then. At a fundamental level the circulatory system works because it can stabilize itself, thanks to the interplay between CO and CVP.

## IS THIS VENTRICLE NECESSARY?

Before leaving our model, let's return to it one more time. Let's ask, would this work for us? Do we really need a right heart? The pulmonary circulation is, after all, a low-resistance system (total pulmonary resistance is only 10% as great as total systemic resistance.) The left ventricle should have no trouble handling this small increase.

Without a right ventricle the capacitance or storage function of the circulatory system would be markedly increased. It would be the total of the systemic venous system plus the pulmonary arterial system. (To picture this better, think of it as a big "portal system" with the systemic microcirculation followed by a large venous system, in turn followed by the pulmonary capillary bed. Then would come the pulmonary veins.) The pressure difference between the systemic veins and the pulmonary veins would be so small that flow through the pulmonary capillaries would be quite slow. That would lower left-heart filling and consequently lower left ventricular output. Raising total blood volume would increase pulmonary blood flow but at the price of markedly increasing systemic venous pressure. This would of course affect capillary function by increasing capillary hydrostatic pressure. We can say therefore that we need a right heart to keep systemic venous pressure and cardiac output in line.

## RATES

We have not yet discussed heart rate. What is the effect of heart rate (HR) on CO? It would seem that the answer is simple: the higher the HR, the greater the CO; the lower the HR, the lower the CO. After all, cardiac output (CO) equals heart rate (HR) times stroke volume (SV). But it is, of course, more complex than that. Change in heart rate can affect the other three factors. With rapid heart rate can come shorter filling time with reduced preload. If increased heart rate increases CO, arterial pressure can be altered, thereby altering afterload. And increased heart rate can increase myocardial contractility. So what really happens?

Generally, at lower heart rates (between 50 and 100), CO goes up as heart rate increases. At more rapid heart rates (between 100 and 180), cardiac output continues to increase but more slowly (a smaller increase in CO with each increment of rising HR). At heart rates above 200, cardiac output falls because filling time is so curtailed. These ranges are certainly approximate and vary among individuals. They also vary in individuals with changes in their physiologic state.

Let's now take up question two: how does this system perform? One way to gain understanding of how a well-regulated system works is to disturb it and see how it responds and how it tries to restore itself to steady state.

## HEMORRHAGE

Severe hemorrhage is, of course, a marked perturbation of the circulatory system. It is reasonable to think that bleeding -- from childbirth or traumatic injury -- has not been a rare occurrence in our evolutionary history so it is also reasonable to expect that we have inherited naturally selected compensatory responses to it. These compensatory responses and their limitations afford insights into circulatory system regulation.

Hemorrhage leads to decreased cardiac output and decline in blood pressure. Because there is less blood to pump, fall in venous return is the primary event. The baroreceptors pick up this fall in pressure and respond by stimulating sympathetic discharge and inhibiting parasympathetic activity. As a result heart rate and myocardial contractility increase, and arteries and arterioles constrict. Arteriolar vasoconstriction is widespread, reducing flow chiefly to striated skeletal muscle and to the gut. With continued or increased low blood pressure, circulation to the kidneys is reduced. There is little or no increase in resistance in the cerebral or coronary vasculature (resistance may even be decreased). Note that this means that the reduced cardiac output is redistributed preferentially to the brain and heart. There is also increased venous constriction reducing venous compliance and recruiting blood volume usually "stored" there.

Baroreceptor response is maximum by the time mean arterial pressure has dropped to 60 mm Hg. Chemoreceptors responding to low oxygen can further increase sympathetic discharge, however.

When arterial pressure falls still more, cerebral ischemia (low blood flow) stimulates even greater sympathetic discharge to the adrenal medulla. (This has already occurred to a lesser degree due to previous sympathetic activity.) More epinephrine and norepinephrine are released into the circulation.

Because arterial and venous blood pressures are down, capillary hydrostatic pressure is also reduced. This allows tissue fluid to be absorbed into the circulation. From this source, as much as 1 liter of fluid an hour can augment the circulating fluid volume.

In addition to catecholamines released from the adrenal medulla, other vasoconstrictors are produced. Vasopressin is released from the posterior pituitary in response to low circulating fluid volume, sensed by the baroreceptors and atrial stretch receptors. The reflex arc carrying this information goes first to the central nervous system medulla and then on to the hypothalamus. Of particular interest is that the decrease in perfusion of the kidneys leads to increase secretion of renin, which leads to an increase in the circulating vasoconstrictor angiotensin.

The kidneys retain sodium and water in response to decreased perfusion, increased vasopressin, and increased aldosterone release (the latter caused by angiotensin).

Despite all these efforts to reestablish the circulation, hemorrhage may be too severe to be survived. In an otherwise healthy person, the loss of 5% to 10% of blood volume is not much of a problem. Loss of 20% is manageable. At 30% and certainly 40% the situation is dicey and requires timely treatment with transfusion. If severe low cardiac output has gone on too long, death ensues even if blood and fluids are transfused.

Herein lies the problem. The circulatory system's efforts to maintain blood flow to the most vital and sensitive organs -- the brain and the heart -- come at a cost. Shunting blood, already in short supply, away from skeletal muscle, the gut, and the kidneys, causes increasing acidity throughout the body (acidosis). Those tissues getting too little oxygen turn, if they can, to anaerobic metabolism, generating lactic acid that diffuses into the bloodstream. Acidosis reduces heart performance and interferes with metabolism generally. The endothelium, when deprived of oxygen and nutrients, malfunctions and may cause diffuse blood clotting often followed by widespread fibrinolysis. Bacterial products from the intestinal tract, chiefly endotoxins which are normally removed by the liver, get through into the general circulation because liver function is depressed. Endotoxin throughout the circulation stimulates nitric oxide synthase to make nitric oxide. The result is marked vasodilatation and circulatory collapse. The brain, assaulted by acidosis, toxins, and lack of nutrients and oxygen, can no longer respond with sympathetic stimulation. So even though the circulatory system's initial responses were perhaps its best choices, the costs can become so great that death may be inevitable and even hastened.

The reactions to mild to moderate hemorrhage that may improve survival have been selected for in the course of evolution. They are by definition compensatory. If some of these same reactions had a detrimental effect on those of our ancestors who suffered severe shock -- so severe as to likely end in death -- they were maintained anyway. From a population standpoint they were still advantageous responses. To the individual for whom present day medical intervention, like blood transfusions and administration of oxygen, is available, some of these responses can jeopardize recovery.

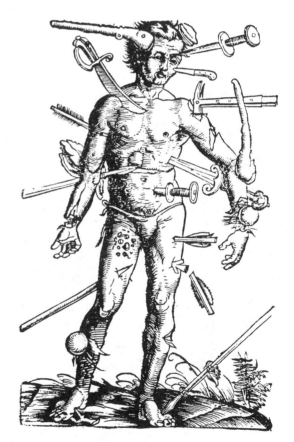

This figure, described as "traditional wound man," dates from the 12th century. It is clearly a catalogue of assaults, any one of which could lead to the circulatory system responses just discussed. Today, of course, we can employ weapons which are both more sophisticated and more effective.

# DISEASES

## 9

---

## REVIEW

How about a short version of Lecture 8?

The circulatory system functions as a unit in large part because cardiac output and central venous pressure (preload) stabilize each other. Each is subject to other influences. Heart rate, myocardial contractility, and afterload help set cardiac output; and blood volume and the amount of venous and arteriolar sympathetic activity help determine central venous pressure.

When the system is stressed by hemorrhage, all its parts working together try to restore its steady state. This effort is often successful unless the insult is too great. Then bad things happen, and are sometimes made even worse by the system's good efforts.

Incidentally, later we will have a chance to see how the circulatory system responds to a happier challenge: exercise.

Is Lecture 9 about more bad things? Some bad, some good. It's about the circulatory system's adaptation to certain disease states.

---

This is not a book about diseases of the circulatory system or of its components. We can, however, add to our understanding and appreciation of how it all works if we look at what happens when something in it goes wrong. How does the circulatory system try to continue to meet its obligation to the body and to all its cells even when it is challenged by problems within its own ranks? With that question in mind we will consider three kinds of circulatory system malfunctions -- heart failure, hypertension, and atherosclerosis.

## HEART FAILURE

The condition heart failure sounds quite dreadful. What is it? When the *circulatory system cannot fully perform* its basic function of providing oxygen and nutrition to and removing carbon dioxide and metabolic waste products from the cells of the body *and it is the heart's fault* -- that is heart failure. Put another way, heart failure occurs when cardiac output is inadequate to meet the body's metabolic needs.

This, of course, can and does occur and for many reasons. If we think about the things that affect cardiac output -- heart rate, myocardial contractility, preload, and afterload -- we can figure that a problem that chronically adversely affects any one or any combination of these factors can stress the heart beyond its capacity to do its job.

One of the most common reasons for cardiac failure is the loss of a piece of heart muscle from a heart attack. When somewhere in the coronary circulation an artery is plugged or critically narrowed, the muscle downstream is deprived of the blood it needs to survive. Because cardiac myocytes cannot divide and replace cells, that piece of heart is lost. The death of tissue resulting from loss of its blood supply is called *infarction*, so this kind of episode is a myocardial infarction. Over time the area of infarction is replaced by scar tissue, but the heart has lost some of its contractility.

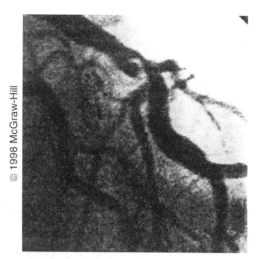

Here is a picture of a left anterior descending coronary artery with a big flap-like plaque. Obviously, this is the kind of narrowing which can lead to infarction of heart muscle tissue.

Another common cause of heart failure is overload from hypertension, chronic high blood pressure. Hypertension produces high afterload, which can eventually tax the heart beyond its limits.

Heart valve abnormalities can over burden the heart in ways that depend on the valve involved and on its specific defect. For example, if the aortic valve (between the left ventricle and aorta) is leaky, then blood from the aorta reenters the left ventricle during

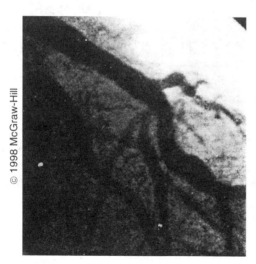

This second picture shows the vessel now totally open. The plaque has been removed by a tiny cutting device on the end of a catheter.

diastole. There is too much preload. If the aortic valve is tight and narrow, the left ventricle has to work hard to push blood out through it. There is too much afterload.

Abnormalities of heart rhythm can reduce cardiac output and cause heart failure. If the pacemaking cells or other parts of the conducting system are faulty, the heart may beat too fast, too slow, or too irregularly.

What happens when the heart "fails"? Because the heart is in fact two pumps, one of the two (left or right) may bear the brunt of whatever insult has created the excess burden, and so may fail more than the other. Thus we hear about "left" or "right" heart failure. In left heart failure, the left ventricle may not be able to keep up and blood backs up into the lungs. In right heart failure, the right ventricle may not be able to handle the amount of blood it receives and blood backs up in the systemic venous system. Certainly both pumps may be affected, and in fact eventually both usually are. Heart failure comes in all degrees of severity. Cardiac output may be inadequate only during significant exercise and be quite satisfactory at rest. On the other end of the spectrum is severely insufficient cardiac output, even when the affected person is at rest in bed.

Whatever the cause, location, or severity of the defect in output, the heart and the rest of the circulatory system -- indeed the rest of the body -- try to make up for it. They all try to adjust and compensate. From early on there is an increase in autonomic sympathetic activity. Cardiac output is encouraged by an increase in both contractility and heart rate from enhanced beta sympathetic activity. Decreased parasympathetic activity also contributes to an increase in heart rate. Vasoconstriction from increased alpha sympathetic discharge helps maintain blood pressure in the face of the tendency for the cardiac output to be reduced. With vasoconstriction, blood flow is maintained to the brain and heart and is reduced to the kidneys, skin, skeletal muscles, and gut. The alpha sympathetic activity also "stiffens" the veins, reducing compliance and enhancing venous return. Circulating blood volume goes up due to stimulation of the renin-angiotensin-aldosterone system. Also vasoconstriction of renal arteries contributes to water retention. The vasopressin (antidiuretic hormone) level is increased, further raising blood volume. The increase in renin release leads to an elevated angiotensin level, which of course contributes to vasoconstriction.

But wait a minute. We have seen all this before. This is what happens when cardiac output goes down because of hemorrhage. This is also the response to circulatory system failure when it is *not* caused by any heart problem.

The body's response to cardiac failure is to try to stabilize the situation by improving pump performance through increased sympathetic drive and volume expansion. Cardiac failure looks and feels to the body like trauma and blood loss, so that is its response paradigm. It is not hard to see why this path of compensation proves to be maladaptive. Cardiac failure is almost always the result of a chronic ongoing problem, not an acute one. Moreover, much of the task of compensation is assigned to the heart, which already has a problem that has made it the weak link.

For starters, vasoconstriction increases afterload and can aggravate the cardiac output shortfall. Increased blood volume augments preload. This ventricular dilating effect can increase the work of contraction and can stretch cardiac sarcomeres to the point of diminishing contractility. And increased heart rate and myocardial contractility from beta stimulation increases the energy demands of the failing heart.

Armed with this information, how would you go about treating heart failure? Of course, if you could do something direct to solve a particular problem like replacing or repairing a defective valve, you would do that. But assuming that the cause of the problem is not so amenable to being fixed, how would you modify those compensatory responses of the body that have become maladaptive?

In the early days, treatment was developed empirically. If something was tried and seemed to help, it was used. Understanding how it worked came later as did efforts to base treatment on understanding of the deranged physiology. For many years treatment for heart failure was limited to two kinds of medicine: digitalis and diuretics.

*Digitalis* has an interesting and in many ways illustrative history. In 1785 William Withering, an English physician, published "An Account of the Foxglove and Some of Its Medical Uses with Practical Remarks on Dropsy and Other Diseases." Foxglove, or *Digitalis purpurea*, is a beautiful plant whose purple flowers look like fingers. Dr. Withering found that its leaves were effective in treating his patients with dropsy. Dropsy, a word derived from hydrops, which refers to water, is the same thing as congestive heart failure. As cardiac failure is very often associated with severe fluid excess,

with leg swelling and lung congestion, it is really best known as congestive heart failure. While digitalis leaf was still being prescribed not many years ago, today a more standardized compound, digoxin, is most common. Even this pure drug has a narrow margin of safety -- there is not much difference between the therapeutic dose and the harmful dose. The reason for this is apparent when we see how digoxin and its cousins work (or at least one of the ways they work).

These drugs poison the $Na^+$, $K^+$-ATPase system, the sodium pump. This causes accumulation of intracellular sodium, interfering with the ability of the sodium/calcium exchanger to bring more sodium into the cell. As a result the exchanger cannot extrude calcium from the cell. With high intracellular calcium, myocyte contraction is enhanced. So digoxin improves myocardial contractility. With the improvement in cardiac output, those forces that increase blood volume by retaining fluid are reduced. With less fluid accumulation in the lungs and other tissues and organs, the symptoms of heart failure are diminished. The way digitalis works seems marginal; that it works at all seems pretty lucky. For years, however, it has been one of the cornerstones of treatment.

*Diuretics* are medications that induce the kidneys to put out sodium and water -- that is, to make an excess of urine. This helps to get rid of the excess fluid in the body. Shortness of breath and leg swelling improve. The congestion of heart failure is reduced.

Other treatments for heart failure are more recent. Drugs are used that relax arteriolar smooth muscle. These vasodilators help to reduce peripheral resistance and thereby reduce afterload. Drugs have been tried that either increase the formation of intracellular cyclic adenosine monophosphate (cAMP) or interfere with its breakdown, all in an effort to enhance myocardial contractility.

The problem with almost all these treatments -- the empirical ones and the scientifically derived ones -- is that, even if they reduce symptoms, they do not prolong life. The average life expectancy in patients with moderate heart failure is less than 5 years. This often remains true if they are treated with medicines that reduce preload or that reduce afterload, or that increase myocardial contractility. In fact, some of the treatments such as phosphodiesterase inhibitors, given to reduce the breakdown of myocyte cAMP, proved to increase mortality.

Why is it that these treatments only relieve

symptoms at best, despite their apparent promise, and are not beneficial in the long term? The answer is "remodeling": in heart failure, a progressive maladaptive change in heart muscle contractility. Here again we are talking about a useful, beneficial capability gone awry. If called on to meet an increasing demand, the heart can become stronger. It can lay down new sarcomeres in its myocytes. Sarcomeres can be added in two ways. They can be laid down in series -- that is, end to end. And they can be laid down in parallel -- that is, side by side. When they are added in series there is no real change in force generated but there is an increase in speed of contraction. Conversely, when sarcomeres are added in parallel arrangement, there is an increase in force generated but no change in speed of contraction.

This hypertrophy of the cells increases the mass of myocardial tissue with enlargement of ventricular diastolic cavity size and increase in ventricular wall thickness. These changes enhance cardiac peak performance. These are the hearts of elite athletes, those who participate in vigorous, prolonged physical activity. Note that there is no increase in the number of cells (hyperplasia). There is only an increase in the size of cells (hypertrophy), but with proportional increases in both their length and width because the new sarcomeres are added both in series and in parallel.

What causes this physiologic remodeling? This is not known but there must be a change in gene expression that leads to protein synthesis, allowing new sarcomeres to be assembled. This whole adaptive process must have been evolutionarily beneficial.

This is probably how the remodeling of heart failure begins, as an adaptive process. In heart failure, however, the increased demand that leads to remodeling is mercilessly unrelenting. There are no periods of normal resting demand, which the elite athlete's heart experiences. Almost from the outset the remodeling response to cardiac failure is harmful.

Take, for example, events that not infrequently occur after a heart attack, even a fairly small one with little immediate reduction in heart performance. The infarcted area of heart muscle undergoes thinning as the dead cells are replaced with scar tissue. Surrounding this is a zone of tissue that is not lost but rather is impaired and has diminished contractility. Viable remaining myocytes undergo hypertrophy with new sarcomeres laid down in series and in parallel but with greater increase in cellular length than in the width. Contractile ventricular wall thickness may in-

crease, but also there is apt to be an increase in chamber diameter -- that is, chamber dilatation. Slippage of myocytes occurs, exaggerating the tendency to dilatation of the ventricle. This dilatation increases the energy required for systole. A smaller proportion of the blood that has filled the left ventricle during diastole is pumped out with each beat (a reduction in ejection fraction). Over time there is progressive change in ventricular structure, and deterioration of its function leading to worsening heart failure.

This kind of hypertrophy is called eccentric hypertrophy and we do know something about its causes. Many of the substances produced in increased amounts in response to cardiac failure -- in fact, just about everything we have talked about -- are promoters of eccentric hypertrophy. Norepinephrine, angiotensin, endothelin, and increased ventricular wall stress all feed into signaling mechanisms that activate kinases, which turn on the enzymes that promote the growth factors that cause remodeling.

It is not surprising then that drugs that reduce angiotensin do have long-term benefit in cardiac failure. Most of them are in the category of angiotensin-converting enzyme (ACE) inhibitors. They block the conversion of angiotensin I to angiotensin II. Not only do ACE inhibitors cause vasodilatation and reduce afterload, but they interfere with ventricular remodeling. Apparently as a result, they do reduce the mortality rate in patients with cardiac failure.

Even more interesting is the use of drugs that block cardiac beta receptors. In the past these beta-blockers were thought to be an improper and even dangerous treatment for cardiac failure. After all, why give something that would tend to further reduce cardiac output? And it is true that a beta-blocker does reduce left ventricular ejection function in patients with cardiac failure and can cause worsening symptoms -- for a few days. After several months of treatment, ejection fraction improves, symptoms improve, and life can be prolonged. The beta-blocker has interfered with remodeling.

What about old, venerable digitalis? Does it really do any good beyond an initial boost in myocardial contractility? There have been some long-standing doubts about its efficacy, but now digitalis has been shown to help relieve symptoms from cardiac failure and not to worsen its long-term outlook. It is not known at this time whether it improves survival in patients with heart failure. It may or it may not. If digitalis does prolong life it must be through a mode of action other than interfering with the sodium pump. One possibility would be the sensitizing effect of digitalis on baroreceptors, which results in a reduction of sympathetic activity and an increase in parasympathetic activity from the central nervous system.

There are other aspects of remodeling that tend to cast it in the paradigm of inflammation and wound healing. We can think of this pattern of response as the body's effort to restore and to heal itself. These are the next steps beyond the initial responses to events perceived as trauma and blood loss.

You recall that in inflammation, cell-to-cell communication is carried out by cytokines, proteins that instruct and stimulate cells to action. One of these cytokines is tumor necrosis factor (TNF). One form, TNF-α, is elevated in cardiac failure, and in fact is produced by the failing human heart. This cytokine induces hypertrophy but it also causes fibrosis (the formation of scar-like tissue) in heart muscle. It is also one of the factors that causes heart cells to self-destruct, a process known as apoptosis. Remember, cardiac myocytes are irreplaceable. It is possible then that drugs that counter TNF would be useful in treating cardiac failure.

Apoptosis can also be induced by norepinephrine and angiotensin, so here may be another reason that beta-blockers and ACE inhibitors cause long-term benefits. In addition it has recently been shown that blocking the action of aldosterone can reduce the process of myocardial fibrosis in heart failure.

Another kind of hypertrophy often occurs in hearts subjected to hypertension. Here, new sarcomeres are laid down mostly in parallel. The wall thickness of the left ventricle is increased, often with little change in chamber size. This pattern is termed concentric hypertrophy. There is some benefit from this because increasing the ventricular wall thickness does reduce wall stress. (The reason for this is based on a corollary of Laplace's law.) However, the same kind of progressive deterioration of cardiac function can occur here that we see in eccentric hypertrophy. Moreover, this situation can create a special set of problems. With a thickened wall the ventricle is stiffer. It has less compliance not only because of reduced elastic recoil but, more importantly, because of relative energy starvation. This means that there is less recoil during diastole and a slower rate of relaxation. The result is decreased diastolic filling. Treatment for this so-called diastolic dysfunction has to date been disappointing.

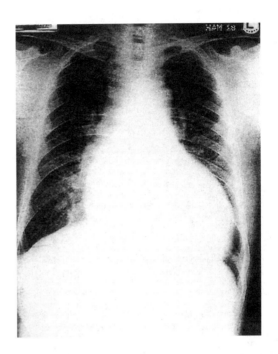

Here is an example of concentric left ventricular hypertrophy due to severe hypertension. Compare the width of this heart to that of the normal heart below.

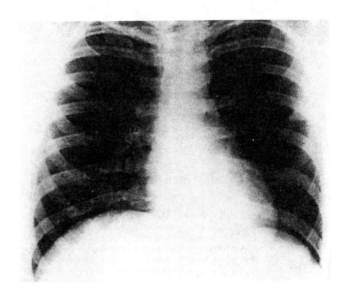

In summary, heart failure is a progressive decline in heart function started when the heart is damaged or otherwise chronically burdened. Sensing a problem the body tries to fix it but the tools it uses don't fit. The body uses them anyway, often making things worse. Evolution, it turns out, never provided the right tools. For our ancestors, Nature in applying its selective judgments had little patience with chronic disease.

## HYPERTENSION

The range of possible blood pressures in human beings is a continuum. How then do we decide at what point one's blood pressure is too high? When does it cross the line and become unacceptable? Perhaps hypertension is a bit like obscenity, as one Supreme Court justice described it, saying, "we'll know it when we see it."

Well, not exactly. The fact is that we define persisting blood pressure of 140/90 or higher as hypertension. This is not an altogether arbitrary choice because it is at this level of 140/90 that the risks of high blood pressure begin to emerge. The risks -- for stroke, heart failure, myocardial infarction, and kidney disease -- then increase as blood pressure increases. At 140/90 it is worth intervening with treatment to try to lower the pressure. Of course, treatment does not always mean medicine. All people with persisting blood pressure elevation require weight normalization, salt restriction, and regular exercise. Sometimes these are all that is needed for mild hypertension.

What then can we learn about the circulatory system from studying this particular problem? For starters we can learn that there are certainly many ways that sustained high blood pressure can come about. And we can sharpen our appreciation and understanding of the complexity of blood pressure controlling mechanisms.

Perhaps the first thing we can learn is that, most of the time, the reason a specific person has hypertension cannot be determined. As many as one-fourth of the adult population in the United States has elevated blood pressure and most of these people have what has long been called *essential hypertension* -- that is, hypertension of unknown cause. This classification no doubt will eventually become smaller as various causal molecular mechanisms are defined. For now, however, we can only say that essential hypertension is characterized by high peripheral vascular resistance due to increased arteriolar smooth muscle tone. This ultimately comes down to too much calcium in the cytoplasm of the smooth muscle cells. Think of all the possibilities -- or at least of some that we know: excessive sympathetic nervous system activity; too much angiotensin or endothelin; too little nitric acid; abnormal G protein signaling inside the cell; and on and on.

In essential hypertension there is not only increased arteriolar tone but also increased venular tone. This ends up reducing the capacity of the venous sys-

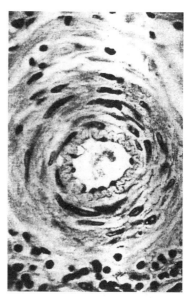

This small artery, subjected to hypertension, has smooth muscle cells in its media which are too large in size and too many in number.

tem. As a result there is a shift of body fluid from inside the circulatory system to the interstitial "compartment." The arteries in hypertension, subjected to higher pressure, increase in wall thickness. This is due to hypertrophy of smooth muscle cells and also to proliferation of these cells. Responding to increased wall stress, smooth muscle cells make some of the growth factors associated with new vessel formation. Angiotensin when elevated also stimulates cell growth. Although this wall thickening helps relieve wall stress, it perpetuates the elevated resistance by reducing the vessel lumen.

Sometimes the underlying cause of hypertension can be defined. Very often this is associated with an increase in a salt-retaining hormone like aldosterone. Here the result is an elevated blood volume instead of a contracted one.

One illustrative example of definable, potentially curable hypertension occurs in an unusual condition known as coarctation (from the Latin word meaning "pressed together") of the aorta. Here, there is a discrete congenital narrowing of the aorta. The narrowed section is usually in the chest, in that part of the aorta after it turns downward. This constriction creates additional resistance. Blood pressure above the narrowing is elevated, and below it is significantly lower than normal. Also only the arteries above the constriction, distended during early systole, contribute to the hydraulic filtering effect. As a result, overall arterial compliance is reduced and pulse pressure is increased, pushing the systolic blood pressure especially high. Hypertension in this condition of coarctation of the aorta is further aggravated by relatively low blood flow to the kidneys. This results in release of renin and the ultimate elevation of angiotensin and aldosterone as well as catecholamines in the blood. This hypertension can usually be cured by surgically correcting the aortic defect.

Hypertension is usually not thought to bring immediate risk. As a rule the adverse consequences of high blood pressure become manifest over time. However hypertensive crises can occur. This uncommon emergency is most often seen in a person whose high blood pressure is already poorly controlled and whose norepinephrine or angiotensin blood levels abruptly increase for some reason. Diastolic blood pressure may be 130 mm Hg or higher. At this level the autoregulating mechanisms in the brain circulation are overwhelmed. The small arterioles are essentially blown open and excessive blood flows to the brain. The result is brain swelling and even hemorrhage. This severe hypertension also damages blood vessels elsewhere. It can cause arterial wall tearing in the aorta; it can damage endothelial cells triggering diffuse blood clotting; it can cause acute cardiac failure by exerting an enormous afterload.

Overall, the risks of hypertension are proportional to its severity and its duration. Let's turn to a frequent complication of hypertension, atherosclerosis.

## ATHEROSCLEROSIS

Atherosclerosis is a word that was coined about one hundred years ago. It is a combination of two words -- *arteriosclerosis*, which literally means hardening of arteries, and *atheroma*, which is the term for the plaque of lipid-containing material that can occur in the intima of an artery. (At the risk of being too vivid, I have to add that the root word of "atheroma" is the Greek word αθηρη, which means gruel.) So atherosclerosis is a process of arterial hardening with narrowing and deformity caused by plaques containing fatty material. It looks like the drawing below.

Right away we are locked onto the idea that this is all a problem of fatty material plugging up vessels. And everyone knows that high blood fats, especially cholesterol, increase the risk of atherosclerosis. Almost everyone knows there is good cholesterol (high-density lipoprotein, HDL) and bad cholesterol (low-density lipoprotein, LDL).

This process is often visualized as globules of

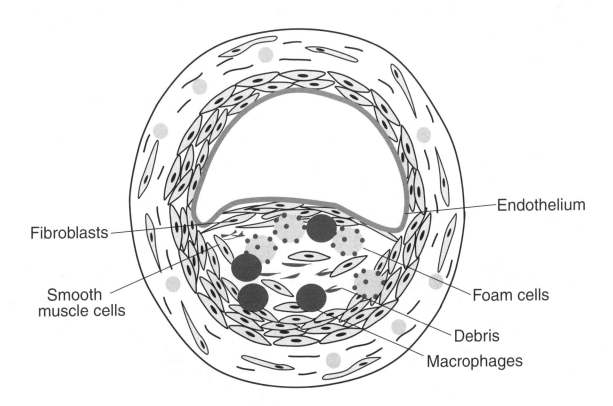

LDL cholesterol floating around in the blood, sticking to the sides of arteries like sludge and gumming up the works. Dispel that picture and let us start over by discussing what LDL and HDL mean.

LDLs are relatively large particles that transport lipids through the plasma. Lipids are water insoluble and have to be packaged into a form that doesn't just separate out. So LDLs are a group of relatively large (large in size, low in density) spheres. Although these are large, compared to other lipoproteins, they are still very small, with diameters averaging 230 angstrom units (2.3 millionths of a centimeter). The outer layer consists of molecules like those we saw in plasma membranes -- only here there is a single layer with water soluble heads to the outside and their lipid soluble tails on the inside. In addition in this outer shell there are cholesterol molecules and special proteins called apolipoproteins. These apolipoproteins interact with enzymes and receptors on cells to move the spheres or their contents in and out of cells. Inside the spheres are the water-insoluble molecules -- chiefly cholesterol esters (cholesterol attached to fatty acids) and some triglycerides (glycerol linked to fatty acids).

HDLs are denser, smaller spheres. Their average diameters are less than half those of LDLs. They have different apolipoproteins on the outside but also have mainly cholesterol esters inside. There are, in fact, other lipoproteins, each with its own mix of lipid cargo, density, size, and apolipoproteins.

These lipoproteins then circulate in the blood and provide a way to get lipophilic molecules to and from cells. Much of this traffic goes through the liver. Remember that fat molecules are vital to the body. Cholesterol is a key precursor for constituents of bile, for many hormones (like aldosterone), and for parts of cell structures. Fatty acids are important sources of energy for many tissues, including those of the heart.

Why then is LDL bad and why is HDL good? One answer is that LDLs transport cholesterol esters to tissues like arteries and HDLs transport lipids away from those arteries to the liver. If there is proportionately too much LDL and too little HDL, then the balance of traffic is toward the arteries. Because cholesterol is not very soluble it builds up in the arteries, making atheromas. This is one explanation of atherosclerosis, and it may even be partly right. But it is flawed by the proposition inherent in its name -- that atherosclerosis is simply a disease of lipid accumulation. The more complete explanation, as it is now coming into focus, is that atherosclerosis is an inflammatory disease.

The lesions of atherosclerosis are found chiefly in large and medium-sized arteries and can cause, by reducing or blocking blood flow, injury and even infarction of tissues -- especially those of the heart, the brain, or the legs. The first step in formation of these lesions is an injury to the arterial endothelium causing it to malfunction. There are probably many things that can deliver the injury, and each usually acts persistently over many years.

LDL, modified by oxidation, is one very likely culprit. Macrophages (tissue monocytes) ingest this LDL in an effort to protect the endothelium. These glutted cells are described as foam cells. Collections of them in arteries form fatty streaks, which are often seen even in the vessels of children. HDL may exert its beneficial effect by interfering with macrophage uptake of oxidized LDL. Once inside the macrophages the LDL continues to push the inflammatory process, however.

Hypertension has inflammation-promoting effects in arteries. Angiotensin, often elevated in hypertension, promotes growth factors that contribute to atheroma progression.

Cigarette smoking promotes atherosclerosis. Which ones among the multitude of toxins produced by smoking make free radicals (and thus cause ongoing endothelial injury) is not clear. Perhaps a better question is, which do not?

Homocysteine can be toxic to endothelial cells. Hereditary diseases of homocysteine metabolism that result in high blood levels of this amino acid can cause severe atherosclerosis even in childhood. Lesser blood level elevations in people without the genetic disease are associated with increased risk to atherosclerosis.

Infection of endothelial cells is an interesting possible cause of atherosclerosis. Two likely suspects, *Chlamydia pneumoniae* and herpesvirus, have been charged but have not yet been convicted.

Whatever the source, once injured, the endothelial cells initiate inflammation by secreting cytokines, some of which recruit monocytes and lymphocytes by inducing specific adhesion molecules on endothelial cell surfaces. In an effort to get rid of or at least to isolate the injurious agent, the artery perpetuates an inflammatory response that can ultimately lead to thickening of the arterial wall. Cytokines and growth factors induce smooth muscle cell migration and proliferation as well as fibrous tissue formation. The result is a thick firm plaque. At first, compensatory dilatation keeps the vessel lumen size stable. However, as the activated inflammatory cells continue their efforts against a persisting foe, the inflamed area enlarges. The advanced plaque ultimately becomes a core of lipid and inflammatory cells covered by a fibrous cap, all of which intrudes into the lumen of the artery, altering blood flow. Furthermore, the fibrous cap may thin out and break open, exposing and releasing clot-promoting factors. With clot formation the vessel may become totally occluded. There is also the risk that small vessels formed within the atheroma itself may bleed, acutely enlarging the plaque.

Atherosclerosis is another example of an imperfect response to an ongoing stress or insult. The insult is varied, the response is inflammation, and the outcome is very often serious.

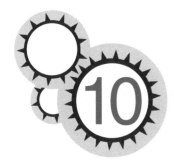

# EXERCISE: THE FINAL KICK

## REVIEW

So what was the good news in Lecture 9?

Congestive heart failure, hypertension, and atherosclerosis are all difficult problems. But all are treatable and more importantly, often preventable. You already know what it takes. Normal weight, good diet low in fat, and no tobacco.

What about exercise? Right! On to Lecture 10.

To end this book with descriptions of maladies and maladaptions would not do. It is fitting that we go out celebrating. So we will finish with a description of one of the circulatory system's wonders: its performance during exercise.

Imagine that you have decided to run a 10-km race, in particular the Bolder Boulder, which is held every year in Boulder, Colorado. So on this bright, cool Memorial Day morning, 42,000 runners are at the starting area. You are waiting in your wave to be called up. There is great excitement, and not a little anticipation. As this group, with you in the middle, starts to surge forward, before you have run a step the cortex of your brain is stimulating your sympathetic system by what is called central command. Not only is there sympathetic discharge, but there is parasympathetic inhibition. Your heart rate is up, as is your cardiac contractility, both increasing cardiac output. Vasoconstriction directs blood away from your skin, kidneys, and gut as well as from muscles that are still inactive. Peripheral resistance and blood pressure are up but moderated by your baroreceptors.

Now your group is moving and you begin to run. Skeletal muscle cells, now active, begin to release potassium and adenosine, and to generate an increasing amount of $CO_2$. Arterioles supplying those muscle cells dilate, as the local flow-regulating mechanisms win out over the neural mechanism that favors vasoconstriction. Blood flow in these arterioles increases, and may go up 15 to 20 times above resting levels during the race. Because the active muscle mass is large, this arteriole dilatation causes a decrease in total peripheral resistance.

As the muscles' terminal arterioles dilate, the number of linked capillaries carrying blood increases. This reduces the diffusion distance between many muscle cells and circulating blood, and it increases the surface area available for exchange of solutes, water, and gases. As the hydrostatic pressure in the capillaries increases, more water and solute are pushed out into the muscle tissue. Tissue pressure rises and more fluid is carried in lymph channels, massaged along by muscle activity.

Active, contracting muscles extract more oxygen, and the venous oxygen saturation goes down. With increased $CO_2$ production and a fall in pH, the oxygen binding by hemoglobin in the capillaries is reduced. Even more oxygen is given up to the muscle cells' mitochondria.

You have settled into a good steady pace. Your heart rate has reached a plateau at about 160 beats a minute, a good deal higher than at rest. Stroke volume is up 25%. In the elite runners of this race the β-adrenergic stimulation of their hearts can result in cardiac output of six to seven times the usual resting level.

As cardiac output goes up and the heart's demand for $O_2$ increases, coronary circulation increases. Blood flow to the brain stays stable. Your increase in cardiac output is matched by increased venous return. This is prompted by increased sympathetic constriction of the veins with associated decreased compliance and reduced capacitance. Venous return is greatly aided by the skeletal muscle pumping action on the veins. It is also aided by deep breathing, which draws more blood during inspiration into the thorax and then on into the right atrium.

Sensing rising body temperature from your work, your brain's hypothalamus effects dilatation of skin arterioles and opening of arteriovenous shunts there. Heat loss is facilitated but your body temperature remains slightly elevated. You are sweating. This causes fluid loss and a decrease in blood volume. Hydrostatic pressure in the capillaries decreases. Fluid loss into muscle tissue goes down and may reverse so that fluid is brought back into the capillaries. Despite this, there is overall reduced blood flow to the kidneys; they make less urine. On your way by the water station at about the halfway point you grab a cup.

Central venous pressure doesn't change much as you complete block after block of the course, so there is not much change in preload. Only at maximal exercise is there some increase in end-diastolic volume, another factor in pushing cardiac output up.

Despite reduction in total peripheral resistance, cardiac output is so increased that arterial blood pressure has risen, though not much. This is abetted by the sympathetic activity that maintains vasoconstriction in relatively inactive tissues. This sympathetic activity is not only from central command but also from reflexes that originate in contracting muscle. For additional sympathetic boost, the adrenal gland releases epinephrine and norepinephrine from its medulla. Even though your mean arterial blood pressure is up only slightly, your pulse pressure is up because of the increase in stroke volume.

Now you are near the stadium. You hear the crowd cheering. You push the pace to finish with a kick but wisely you don't overdo it.

If you did push to the point of exhaustion, your compensating mechanisms would begin to fail. A higher heart rate would start to reduce stroke volume (by cutting into filling time) to the point that cardiac output would fall. Blood pressure would start to drop. Body temperature would increase because sympathetic vasoconstriction would supersede vasodilation in the skin. The pH would fall further as muscles, not getting enough oxygen, would rely more on anaerobic activity.

You avoided all these problems though. You enter the stadium and soon cross the finish line, in a time befitting your preparation and training. As you slow to a walk, the sympathetic drive to your heart is removed. Your heart rate and cardiac output decrease. Total peripheral resistance remains low until the substances ($K^+$, adenosine, $H^+$) that were causing the local arteriolar effects are cleared. Blood pressure falls and would go below usual levels but is stabilized by your baroreceptors.

It is a good thing you trained for this race for several weeks. The factors that place limits on exercise performance are oxygen delivery to muscles (which is determined chiefly by cardiac output) and oxygen use by skeletal muscle. By training you were able to increase your stroke volume and reduce your total peripheral resistance. You induced lower vascular resistance in the muscles used in running and enhanced their ability to extract oxygen from the blood. If you had trained over a longer period of time you could even have increased the number of capillaries and arterioles in your leg muscles and the mitochondria in those muscles cells.

You ran a good race. Your circulatory system performed very well. And I hope you enjoyed the course.